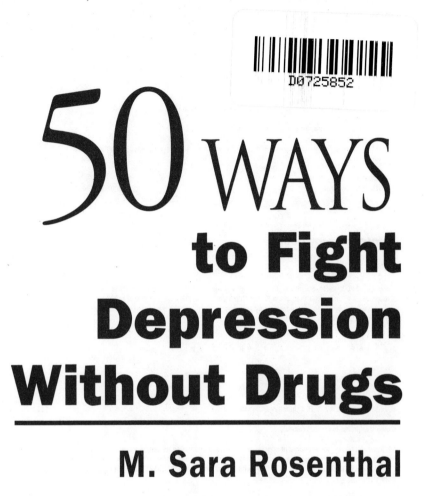

50 WAYS
to Fight
Depression
Without Drugs

M. Sara Rosenthal

Contemporary Books

Chicago New York San Francisco Lisbon London Madrid Mexico City
Milan New Delhi San Juan Seoul Singapore Sydney Toronto

D0725852

Library of Congress Cataloging-in-Publication Data

Rosenthal, M. Sara.
    50 ways to fight depression without drugs / M. Sara Rosenthal.
       p.   cm.
    Includes bibliographical references and index.
    ISBN 0-7373-0557-6
    1. Depression, Mental—Treatment—Popular works.   I. Title: Fifty ways to fight depression
without drugs.   II. Title.

  RC537.R63848   2002
  616.85′2706—dc21
                                   2001053796

Contemporary Books

A Division of The McGraw·Hill Companies

1 2 3 4 5 6 7 8 9 0   DOC/DOC   1 0 9 8 7 6 5 4 3 2

ISBN 0-7373-0557-6

This book was set in Cochin
Printed and bound by R. R. Donnelley—Crawfordsville

Cover design by Jeanette Wojtyla

McGraw-Hill books are available at special quantity discounts to use as premiums and sales promotions, or for use in corporate training programs. For more information, please write to the Director of Special Sales, Professional Publishing, McGraw-Hill, Two Penn Plaza, New York, NY 10121-2298. Or contact your local bookstore.

The purpose of this book is to educate. It is sold with the understanding that the author and publisher shall have neither liability nor responsibility for any injury caused or alleged to be caused directly or indirectly by the information contained in this book. While every effort has been made to ensure the book's accuracy, its contents should not be construed as medical advice. Each person's health needs are unique. To obtain recommendations appropriate to your particular situation, please consult a qualified health care provider.

The herbal information in this book is provided for educational purposes only and is not meant to be used without consulting a qualified health practitioner who is trained in herbal medicine.

This book is printed on acid-free paper.

Contents

Acknowledgments

I wish to thank the following people, whose expertise and dedication helped to lay so much of the groundwork for this book and who have served as advisors on past works on the topic of depression: Debra Lander, M.D., FRCPC, Assistant Professor of Psychiatry, University of Manitoba; Mark Lander, M.D., FRCPC, Associate Professor of Psychiatry, University of Manitoba, and a member of the Mood Disorders Clinic, Health Sciences Centre, Winnipeg, Manitoba; and Sheila Lander, LPN/RN, a psychiatric nurse practitioner, Health Sciences Centre, Winnipeg, Manitoba.

I'd also like to thank Donna Stewart, M.D., FRCP, Lillian Love Chair in Women's Health, University Health Network and University of Toronto; Judith Ross, Ph.D., Clinical Psychologist and Special Lecturer, Department of Psychology, University of Toronto; and Trudo Lemmens, LicIur, LLM (Bioethics), Assistant Professor, Faculty of Law, Department of Molecular Medicine and Microbiology and Department of Psychiatry, and formerly Bioethicist at the Centre for Addiction and Mental Health; and clinical psychologists Sergio Rueda, M.S., and Eliana Cohen, M.S., Ph.D. (candidate), Department of Psychology, York University.

, A number of past medical advisors on previous works also must be thanked: Gillian Arsenault, M.D., CCFP, IBLC, FRCP; Pamela Craig, M.D., FACS, Ph.D.; Masood Kahthamee, M.D., FACOG; Gary May, M.D., FRCP; James McSherry, MB, ChB, FCFP, FCFP, FRCGP, FAAFP, FABMP; Suzanne Pratt, M.D., FACOG; and Robert Volpe, M.D., FRCP, FACP.

William Harvey, Ph.D., LLB, Director, University of Toronto Joint Centre for Bioethics, whose devotion to bioethics has inspired me, continues to support my work, and makes it possible for me to have the courage to question and challenge issues in health care and medical ethics. Irving Rootman, Ph.D., Director, University of Toronto Centre for Health Promotion, continues to encourage my interest in primary prevention and health promotion issues.

Larissa Kostoff, my editorial consultant, worked very hard to make this book come into being. And finally, Claudia McCowan, developmental editor, made many wonderful and thoughtful suggestions to help make this book what it is.

Introduction

Depression, mood swings, and other mood and anxiety disorders cause great suffering to millions of Americans. Indeed, the U.S. Surgeon General recently labeled suicide a major public health problem; mood disorders are clearly the most important factor related to completed suicides.

The majority of people suffering from depression have *unipolar depression*, a mood disorder characterized by one low mood. This is distinct from *bipolar depression*, a mood disorder in which there are two moods—one high and one low. This book will show you ways to modify your lifestyle and reduce stress, which may help prevent the development of unipolar depression; bipolar depression is not discussed.

Unipolar depression is usually caused by life circumstances or situations. For this reason, the term *situational depression* is used by mental health care experts to describe most cases of mild, moderate, or even severe unipolar depression. Situational depression can mean that your depression has been triggered by a life event such as the following:

- Illness
- The loss of a loved one (the relationship may have ended, or a loved one may have died)
- A major life change
- Job loss or change
- Moving

Situational depression can also mean that your unipolar depression has been triggered by the *absence* of change in your life, meaning that you are living in a state of continuous struggle, unhappiness, or stress, and no light appears at the end of the tunnel. Examples of continuous struggle include:

- Chronic illness
- Unhealthy relationships
- Poverty and/or economic worries
- Job stress
- Body image problems, such as feeling fat or unattractive

A third cause of situational depression is when unipolar depression is triggered by an absence of resolution regarding past traumas and abuses you suffered as a child or younger adult. These could be any of the following:

- Sexual abuse or incest
- Violence
- Rape
- Emotional abuse

If you've experienced situational depression in the past, this book will show you some ways to help prevent future episodes without having to use antidepressants. If you've never experienced depression but are concerned that you are at risk, this book will show you ways to reduce, or even eliminate, common stressors that can trigger depression. If you are currently in treatment with a therapist or are taking medication, this book is *not a substitute* for these interventions and should be used as a companion to your existing therapy.

50 Ways to Fight Depression explains the differences between normal emotional responses such as sadness and grief, and what we call depression (Part I). Indeed, you may benefit from knowing that you are simply sad and not clinically depressed; on the flip side, recognizing the signs of depression can help you seek treatment earlier so you can get your life back sooner. This book will also provide you with unique information on the best-known secret to good mental health: passion (Part II). By rediscovering your passion—in all its forms—you can reengage with the world around you, which is your best defense against depression.

There is a strong association between stress and depressive moods; therefore, reducing stress (Part III) is an important way to prevent depression. You may not realize how crucial good physical health is when it comes to staying well emotionally and mentally. Physical activity, good eating habits, and mind-strengthening exercises such as meditation (Part IV) are extremely important to your mental health. Finally, incorporating self-care strategies (Part V) into your daily routine may dramatically reduce current stressors associated with depression.

PART I

Sadness Versus Depression

1. Know the Signs of Sadness

The million-dollar question is: Are you depressed or just sad? Everyone experiences sadness, bad days, and blue moods from time to time. Feeling sad is not the same thing as being depressed. So the first order of business is to define what normal sadness is and how it is distinct from depression.

What exactly is sadness? *Sadness* can be defined as mental anguish or suffering in the absence of any physical pain, such as experiencing the death of a loved one or empathizing with a loved one who is ill. A mother watching her child suffer, for example, is not in any physical pain, but she still suffers and experiences sadness. When we are sad, our emotions are expressed through crying, talking, or thinking continuously about our sorrow. We may find it difficult to sleep, concentrate, and eat. Sadness is characterized by sad feelings—the opposite of the numbness that is the main feature of depression.

The problem for many people in affluent cultures is that often sadness is not triggered by anything obvious. For example, our sadness can develop when we realize our lives or situations are not improving or are even declining. Stagnating (being in a rut) or finding your life is getting worse rather than better are conditions that lead to sadness and suffering. As human beings, once our basic needs (safety, food, shelter, love) are looked after, we are driven toward self-actualization. But when our life circumstances stymie self-actualization or spiritual growth, we suffer and feel sad. The longing for material possessions, money, or an intimate relationship is often just an expression of the desire for self-realization. Later in life, many of us also begin to question our attachments to material possessions and power; as we get older, we begin to see the difference between real needs (such as love, friendship, and respect) and artificial needs (such as money, power, and prestige).

For those of us who like the status quo and our quality of life, sadness and suffering can develop when a life event of some kind threatens that status quo, our sense of our own identity, or our quality of life. The threat can come from an infinite variety of sources, of course, ranging from physical illness to financial hardship.

Sadness Versus Depression

Sadness *lifts*, depression *persists*. That's how you can tell whether you're just feeling sad or are actually depressed. Feelings of sadness and grief (see the following section in this chapter) are definitely common and normal in an infinite variety of circumstances. And, again, the symptoms of sadness often mirror depression: you cry; you can't sleep; you can't eat. But eventually, as time passes and you find yourself going back to your routine, the sadness lifts. You may still be sad or grieving, but you can also enjoy your life and put your sad thoughts on the back burner. That's not to say that the problem disappears, but with the right support you will be able to cope. You may need to talk about your problem or life event to friends or family, but every day gets easier. You can get out of bed and have appreciation for something in life, whether it's a nice day, a funny movie, or a good dessert. When you're depressed, nothing lifts; life gets more difficult, grayer, and bleaker until you begin to feel numb, and what you once found pleasurable no longer interests you. Your ability to function will *decrease* with each passing day when you're depressed, whereas your ability to function will *increase* each day when you're just sad. But the trigger—the event that has caused you to become sad or depressed—is always real, understandable, and legitimate. Never forget that.

What is tricky about the "sadness versus depression" question is that what triggered your sadness can also trigger depression. Again, when the symptoms persist rather than lift, you are not getting better and may need some help. Instead of every day getting better, every day gets worse.

2. Know the Signs of Grieving

One of the most common causes of sadness and suffering is grief. If you're grieving the loss of a loved one, and profound feelings of sadness and an inability to eat, sleep, or concentrate persist beyond three months, your grief may have begun to develop into a full-blown depression. Because women outlive their spouses more often than men do, women tend to suffer from grief more often. About 10 percent of all people who suffer the loss of a loved one require treatment for depression. But certain people are more likely to become depressed after such a loss. Those with a history of depression, those who have lost a relationship of many years, and those who have lost a relationship that was unresolved (creating profound feelings of guilt and regret) are more likely to suffer from depression. When depression is triggered by grief, feelings of low self-worth or inadequacy are likely connected to your loss and coming to the surface.

It's important to remember that you can also grieve for the loss of someone who's still very much alive. When a relationship or friendship ends, your feelings of grief over the loss of that relationship are similar to the grief experienced when someone dies.

For many people, the loss of a pet can create profound feelings of grief. But because of embarrassment over the feelings we have for our pets, many of us are afraid to admit or express our grief in this situation. But pets are real companions who offer unconditional acceptance and love. They may serve as vessels for many emotions that never get released into relationships with other human beings. And people are often guilt-ridden over putting their pets to sleep, which adds another dimension to the grieving.

Grief may have progressed to depression when:

- Your grief persists longer than three months
- You feel like dying or are suicidal
- You are experiencing hallucinations or delusions (for example, you see your loved one or believe he or she is still alive)
- You feel depressed every day and have experienced the symptoms of depression discussed in the next section for more than a month
- You aren't caring for yourself (for example, you're not eating, bathing, and so on)

3. Know the Signs of Depression

Depression is distinct from sadness in that it is a point *beyond* sadness, characterized by a numbness and inability to act. Depression is clinically known as a mood disorder. It's impossible to define what a "normal mood" is, because we all have complex personalities and exhibit different moods throughout a given week or even a given day. But it's not impossible for you to define what a normal mood is for you. You know how you feel when you're functional: you're eating; sleeping; interacting with friends and family; being productive, active, and generally interested in life's daily goings-on. Depression is when you feel you've lost the ability to function for a prolonged period of time, or when you're functioning at a reasonable level for the outside world, but you've lost interest in participating in life.

One bad day, or even a bad week (which will probably still include some "relief time," where you can laugh at or take pleasure in something), from time to time does not indicate that you're depressed. Feeling you've lost the ability to function as you normally do—all day, every day—for a period of at least two weeks may be a sign of depression. The symptoms of depression can vary from person to person, but can include some or all of the following:

- Feelings of sadness and/or "empty mood"
- Difficulty sleeping (usually waking up frequently in the middle of the night)
- A loss of energy and feelings of fatigue and lethargy
- A change in appetite (usually a loss of appetite)
- Difficulty thinking, concentrating, or making decisions
- Loss of interest in formerly pleasurable activities, including sex
- Anxiety or panic attacks
- Obsessive attention to negative experiences or thoughts

- Feelings of guilt, worthlessness, hopelessness, or helplessness
- Restlessness and irritability
- Thoughts about death or suicide (see Section 5 on dealing with such thoughts later in this chapter)

When You Can't Sleep

The typical sleep pattern of a depressed person is to go to bed at the normal time, only to wake up around two in the morning and find that he or she can't get back to sleep. Endless hours are spent watching infomercials to pass the time, or simply tossing and turning, usually obsessing over negative experiences or thoughts. Lack of sleep affects our ability to function and leads to increased irritability, lack of energy, and fatigue. Insomnia by itself is not a sign of depression, but when you look at depression as a package, the inability to fall or stay asleep can aggravate all the other symptoms. In some cases, people who are depressed will oversleep, requiring ten to twelve hours of sleep every night.

When You Can't Think Clearly

Another debilitating feature of depression is finding that you simply can't concentrate or think clearly. You feel scattered, disorganized, and unable to prioritize. This usually hits hardest in the workplace or school, and can severely impair your performance on the job. You may miss important deadlines or meetings, or find you can't focus when you do attend meetings. When you can't think clearly, you can be overwhelmed with feelings of helplessness or hopelessness. "I can't even perform a simple task such as this any-more" may dominate your thoughts, while you become more disillusioned with your dwindling productivity.

Anhedonia: When Nothing Gives You Pleasure

One of the most telling signs of depression is a loss of interest in activities that used to excite you or give you pleasure. This is known as anhedonia, derived from the word *hedonism*. A hedonist is a person who indulges his or her every pleasure without considering (or caring about) the consequences. Anhedonia simply means "no pleasure."

Different people have different ways of expressing anhedonia. For example, you might tell your friends you don't have any desire to do X or Y; you can't get motivated; or X or Y just doesn't hold your interest or attention. You may also notice that the sense of satisfaction from a job well done is simply gone, which is particularly debilitating in the workplace or school. For example, artists (photographers, painters, writers, etc.) may find the passion has gone out of their work.

Many of the other symptoms of depression hinge on this loss of pleasure. One of the reasons weight loss is so common in depression (typically, people may notice as much as a ten-pound drop in their weight) is because food or cooking no longer gives them pleasure. The sense of satisfaction from having a clean home or clean kitchen also may disappear. Therefore, tackling kitchen cleanup in order to prepare food may be too taxing, contributing to a lack of interest in eating.

Of course, gaining weight is also not unusual, and ten pounds in the opposite direction can occur, too. This is often due to poor nutrition as well, because we're not eating properly. We fill up on snack foods or high-calorie, low-nutrient foods because we're not motivated to prepare or eat well-balanced meals. Weight gain also may come from a loss of interest in physical activities—exercising, sports, or a dozen other things that keep us active when we're feeling ourselves.

A loss of interest in sex aggravates matters if we are in a romantic relationship with someone. Again, the decreased desire for sex stems from general anhedonia.

4. Rule Out Biological Causes for Depression

If you're suffering from what appear to be symptoms of depression, see your doctor and be sure to rule out the following physical conditions:

- Chronic fatigue syndrome
- Thyroid disease
- Sleep disorders (such as sleep apnea or narcolepsy)
- Side effects from any medications you're taking
- Hepatitis
- Seasonal depression
- Obesity-related fatigue
- Lyme disease
- Sexually transmitted diseases, including HIV and syphilis
- Anemia (Fatigue is often a symptom of anemia; in women, it can be due to heavy menstrual flow.)

- Allergies (Delayed symptoms of an allergic reaction can be joint aches, pains, eczema, and fatigue. Foods and environmental toxins can be classic triggers.)

Chronic Fatigue Syndrome

Chronic fatigue syndrome (CFS) refers to a collection of ill-health symptoms (not just one or two), the most identifiable of which are fatigue and flulike aches and pains. It wasn't until 1994 that an official definition of CFS was actually published in the *Annals of Internal Medicine*. The Centers for Disease Control and Prevention (CDC) have since published their own list of official symptoms. Although many physicians feel the following list is limited and requires some expansion for accuracy, as of this writing, the official defining symptoms of CFS include:

- A "new" unexplained fatigue. In other words, you previously felt fine and have only noticed in the last six months or so that you're always fatigued, no matter how much rest you get. The fatigue is also debilitating for you; you're not as productive at work, and it interferes with normal social, personal, or academic activities. You've also noticed poor memory or concentration, which affects your activities and performance.

- In addition to this fatigue, you have four or more of the following, which have persisted for at least six months:

Sore throat

Mild or low-grade fever

Tenderness in the neck and underarm area (may be caused by swollen lymph nodes)

Muscle pain (called myalgia)

Pain along the nerve of a joint, without redness or swelling

A strange and new kind of headache you've never had before

Sleep that leaves you unrefreshed (a sign of insufficient amounts of non-REM sleep, as discussed in Part V)

Fatigue, weakness, and general malaise for a good twenty-four hours after you've had even moderate exercise

It is possible you may be diagnosed with a frustrating label called *idiopathic fatigue*, which means that your fatigue is of unknown origin. This is not very helpful, and you should find out why you don't meet CFS criteria if your symptoms persist.

Fibromyalgia Versus CFS

Fibromyalgia is a soft-tissue disorder that causes you to hurt all over—all the time. It appears to be triggered and/or aggravated by stress. If you primarily notice fatigue with general aches and pains, this suggests CFS. If you primarily experience joint and muscle pains accompanied by fatigue, this may be fibromyalgia.

Fibromyalgia is sometimes considered an offshoot of arthritis, and it's often misdiagnosed as rheumatoid arthritis. Headaches, morning stiffness, and an intolerance to cold, damp weather are common complaints when you have fibromyalgia. It's also common to suffer from irritable bowel syndrome or bladder problems with this disorder.

Thyroid Disease

The thyroid gland is responsible for making thyroid hormone, which drives the function of every cell in your body.

If your gland is either overproducing or underproducing this hormone, your energy levels and emotional responses will be greatly affected. When the gland is not making enough thyroid hormone, you suffer from *hypothyroidism*; when it is making too much, you have *hyperthyroidism*. In most cases, autoimmune diseases cause the thyroid gland to malfunction, which means your body produces antibodies that attack the gland.

The most common autoimmune diseases associated with the thyroid are Graves' disease and Hashimoto's disease. Graves' disease results in an overactive thyroid gland, while Hashimoto's disease causes the gland to be underactive. Women suffer from thyroid disorders about ten times more frequently than men and therefore are most often subject to misdiagnosis of a thyroid condition.

Symptoms of thyroid disease come in two groups; the type of symptoms you suffer depends on whether you're hyperthyroid or hypothyroid. If you're hyperthyroid, your body speeds up and becomes overworked. Your heart rate increases; you may lose weight but eat more; you may notice excessive perspiration, an intolerance to heat, irregular periods, and diarrhea. You will also experience many of the same symptoms seen in depression, such as exhaustion (from an overworked physique), insomnia, irritability, restlessness and nervousness, anxiety, and general fatigue (caused by the insomnia).

If you're hypothyroid, your body slows down, creating physical symptoms that include constipation, bloating and fluid retention, a decreased appetite, lack of sex drive, dry hair, dry skin, intolerance to cold temperatures, and irregular periods. The emotional symptoms of hypothyroidism are different: extreme fatigue and lethargy regardless of how much sleep you get, as well as symptoms of depression.

A simple blood test will confirm whether you are hyper- or hypothyroid. Treatment for hyperthyroidism depends on what's causing the gland to be overactive; ultimately, your thyroid gland will probably be chemically "deadened" and you'll be given synthetic thyroid hormone (levothyroxine sodium), which replaces the natural hormone your gland makes. If you have hypothyroidism, a synthetic hormone replenishes or "tops up" your diminished supply. For more information, consult *The Thyroid Sourcebook*, 4th edition, or *The Hypothyroid Sourcebook*.

Seasonal Affective Disorder (SAD)

Many people suffer from seasonal depression, which has more to do with a lack of sunlight than anything else. Seasonal affective disorder is a fairly recent label that was coined in 1987. A person with SAD will notice that during the winter, he or she sleeps too much and eats too much (thereby gaining weight). This person then begins to "wake up" in the spring and can even be slightly euphoric. In short, SAD has many of the features of hibernation—oversleeping and storing up on high fat or carbohydrates for the cold winter. It's "bear and squirrel" behavior in humans, which can be debilitating.

This disorder strikes people in their twenties and thirties, and is seen more often in regions at higher latitudes. Living or working in areas that are light-deprived can also lead to SAD. For example, people who spend weeks or months at a time on submarines exhibit symptoms of SAD.

There is now light at the end of the tunnel—literally—for people who suffer from seasonal depression. If you've been diagnosed with SAD, your practitioner may prescribe light. Often, the "cure" is to re-create the kind of light you'd naturally be exposed to on a nice summer's day. Sitting under your chandelier won't do. You need to be sitting in front of bright, full-spectrum fluorescent or incandescent lights for about 30 to 120 minutes for this to work. It's not necessary to have sunlight or sunlike light. To protect your eyes, the lights are covered with a sheer material. You can get the light you need with a "light box." Just do whatever you like in front of these lights. You'll need to sit close — only about a foot and a half away. For the therapy to work, you need to keep your eyes open, so napping isn't a good thing. (If you prefer to sleep, there is an experimental device known as a dawn simulator that can work while you sleep.) Most people start to feel better within a few days of beginning daily thirty-minute light treatments.

This treatment does come with some side effects: mild headaches or eyestrain are not unusual, and sometimes mild mania (from the production of serotonin) may even occur. In this case, you may feel "high" or slightly euphoric. If you're taking a drug that makes you sensitive to bright light, you are not a good candidate for this therapy. See your doctor for information on purchasing a light box.

Bright light therapy has also been shown to help depression not necessarily related to SAD, but rather to sleep problems involving what's known as circadian rhythm sleep disorders. In this case, light therapy during the day has been shown to help establish proper sleep patterns.

5. Know How to Deal with Suicidal Thoughts

About 40 percent of all people who suffer from depression have thoughts of suicide. You may have hoarded pills, bought a gun, prepared a will, or written a suicide letter. If you're thinking life isn't worth living or have considered acting on such thoughts, doing just one of these things can help:

- Call a friend, family member, therapist, or family doctor right away. Tell this person how you're feeling and say you need help to make it through the moment/hour/day.

- Go directly to a hospital emergency room and seek help from a doctor, nurse, or other health care provider.

- Call a suicide help line, listed in the white pages of your telephone book.

If you live with someone you're afraid may be suicidal, lock away knives, guns, and any other weapons, and empty the medicine cabinets of all medicines. You may need to restrict the person's access to car keys. Then, call 911 and report your concerns; an emergency services team can help get your loved one to the right professional.

6. Understand Who Gets Depressed

More then 19 million Americans over the age of eighteen suffer from some type of depression each year. Depression is the leading cause of disability worldwide, according to a recent study by the World Health Organization, the World Bank, and Harvard University. Nearly twice as many women (12%) as men (7%) are affected by a depressive illness. There are some reasons for this:

- The social conditions for women are often more difficult than they are for men, and women tend to seek help more often than men do.

- Women in their twenties and thirties are at risk for postpartum depression.

- In later life, women often grieve the loss of their spouses or feel socially isolated.

National statistics show that people born after 1940 suffer from depression and other mood disorders more often than those born before that year. But that says much more about the social structure that has emerged since 1940 than it does about people. There is no proof that more people are depressed today than were depressed during, say, the Great Depression (no pun intended). That's because no one studied or "counted" how many people were depressed back then; if someone had, it is likely he or she would have found similar numbers of depressed individuals, given the economic misery of that period.

7. Understand the Causes of Depression

Since most episodes of depression are triggered by life events or circumstances, the causes of depression are different for everyone. In a very general way, the direct answer to the question of what causes depression is: difficult circumstances. Understanding what's "difficult" is akin to understanding pain thresholds. What one person finds difficult, another may not.

What we know is that depression is on the rise — or at least, the diagnosis of depression is on the rise. Not unlike other illnesses or diseases, when there is awareness and "active screening" for a particular condition (in this case, such screening is done through diagnostic criteria listed in the *Diagnostic and Statistical Manual of Mental Disorders, Fourth Edition* [DSM IV], an often-criticized "recipe book" of psychiatric symptoms published by the American Psychiatric Association), there is a rise in the number of cases reported. In other words, when you're looking for something, you'll find it. Of course, not looking for something doesn't mean it isn't there. The question remains: Is it better to seek out depression and treat it, ending unnecessary suffering? Many health care practitioners would answer, "Yes!"

Although there is some agreement among health care providers that depression is a biological state — in that brain chemistry is altered in depressed people — it is unusual for this to occur in the absence of an environmental trigger, meaning a life event or chronic situation. This can be an actual emotional trauma, such as a divorce or death; unresolved traumas from the past that have been buried; repressed anger (a significant contributing factor for many women); stress from the workplace; physical illness; and a million other things. When a life event triggers depression, mental health experts refer to the condition as "situational depression."

Some Depressing Circumstances

It's useful to look at some of the life events that are common triggers of situational depression.

• *Poverty*. Difficulty paying bills and making ends meet leads to feelings of anxiousness, sleeplessness, stress, guilt, irritability, and persistent physical symptoms. And poverty is tiring: many people need to work at two or three jobs in order to survive and cannot afford the conveniences that make life easier. This can lead to fatigue, loss of energy, loss of appetite, and so on. Debt is a new spin on poverty. The poverty is often hidden because people live in seemingly comfortable surroundings even though they have "maxed out" their credit cards to pay the rent in between jobs or contracts; are being harassed by creditors; and are one day away from having their car repossessed. It's important to note that many people in poverty or debt are also the "hidden homeless," even though they are not visible on the streets. Untold numbers camp out on the couches of friends and relatives, looking for employment or a place to live.

• *Workplace stress*. Workplace stress and "desk rage" is rampant. Long hours and commuting takes its toll. See Part III for tips on reducing job stress.

• *Illness*. Chronic illness is a contributing factor in many cases of depression. People living with chronic diseases can experience many of the symptoms associated with depression, such as loss of appetite, sleeplessness, and loss of interest in formerly pleasurable activities. To aggravate matters, medications ranging from chemotherapy to AZT can cause depression.

• *Major life changes*. Moving, changing jobs, having a baby, taking in an ailing parent, and other situations that significantly change your life—even for the better—can trigger depression.

• *Divorce*. The dissolution of a long-term relationship with an intimate partner leads to feelings of grief, sadness, loneliness, isolation, and often financial hardship—all fodder for depression.

8. Understand Why People Get Depressed

When we must change or challenge an old way of being or thinking, depression may be the state that many of us enter to deal with the crisis and hopefully emerge from it more true to ourselves. Whether depression entails a slowdown or a complete halt in our daily life, its symptoms may be necessary for us to reroute or change directions emotionally, so that we can either continue along the road to self-actualization or perhaps discover it for the first time. Self-actualization may or may not lead to greater happiness or fulfillment, however, because many times, ignorance is still bliss.

Greater self-knowledge tends to "burst our bubbles" and tears down walls we've spent years building to protect ourselves. Unfortunately, human beings are driven to the path that leads to greater truth. Whether the truth is forced on us through circumstances that are beyond our control or we (un)consciously set ourselves up to discover it, truth is like a baby: it is born out of pain and suffering. Sometimes, when the pain and suffering are too great, we give ourselves an emotional anesthetic that numbs things for a while and manifests as depression.

Even when depression seems to come out of nowhere, it is the body's and soul's way of getting us to stop and think about our life. Depression invariably comes from somewhere. It may be a state we enter to save ourselves from decisions or actions that can lead to bad consequences. For example, Antti Mattila, M.D., a Finnish researcher who has explored why we get depressed from a philosophical perspective, suggests that the inability to act or communicate has a larger purpose for people at different crossroads in life. When we find our values and goals shifting or stirring, and we're in a state of confusion, often the worst thing we can do is act or make a decision. That period of indecision is valuable because it enables us to stop and reflect.

There may also be a larger purpose to the anxiety and melancholy that accompany the confusion or inaction we experience with depression. For example, the philosopher Kierkegaard believed that periods of depression (which he described as melancholy and angst) are simply part of authentic human existence; in short, a person who never knows melancholy will never know metamorphosis. And he described angst as a sign that one is realizing the field of possibilities that comes from free will. It is a time when a person contemplates past choices or circumstances and thinks about ways to make new choices or change his or her circumstances.

Heidegger, another philosopher, suggests that anxiety is also part of the human experience and an indication that the world (situations, relationships, contacts, etc.) isn't "working" for us anymore, forcing us to reconstruct the world around us.

In other words, when you're in a rut or feel trapped by life's circumstances, sadness and suffering or depression can be your mind's and body's way of saying, "Wake up and change." In this case, the only way to stop the suffering is to change the conditions of your life (as in leaving a job you hate) or at least change the way you view the conditions of your life (as in seeing a layoff as something that has allowed you to go back to school and change professions rather than as a curse). In other words, if you can't change your life, you can still change your perspective on it, which can be a huge life-changing event, even though the conditions of your life remain the same.

9. Understand the Types of Depression

You now understand the difference between sadness, grief, and depression. But what you may not realize is that not all depression is the same. There are many types of depression, each with its own distinguishing symptoms and meaning. Mood disorders are divided into two categories: unipolar (one pole, or "one mood") and bipolar (two poles, or "two moods"). This book deals only with unipolar depression. Someone with a unipolar disorder will have one low, or blue, mood. The following are all considered common unipolar disorders.

Major Depression

The symptoms of depression listed on pages 7–8 refer to major depression, the "cold and flu" for mental health care providers, because it is so common. The more severe the depression, the more numb you may be, making it difficult to feel anything—good or bad—for anyone or anything in your life. This is the kind of depression that most often leads to suicide or suicidal thoughts. And major depression by itself can manifest as a mild, moderate, or severe episode. To confuse matters, the condition discussed in the next section, dysthymia, is often referred to as "mild depression."

Dysthymia

Pronounced *dis-thy-mee-ah*, this is a chronic low mood that manifests as a bad attitude to life. The symptoms are very vague and include an intolerance to stress, or stress "overwhelm"; feelings of dependence toward others; a lack of warm or loving emotions; a desire to run away from life, to give up; sensitivity to criticism; an inability to have fun; constant "grumpy" behavior; a belief that life isn't worth living; a tendency to be overcritical and complain all the time. Even though this probably sounds like a lot of people you know, these symptoms add up to what is considered to be a mild form of depression. Mental health care providers insist that a person with dysthymia is not just someone with a bad or off-putting personality but someone who can be helped. The condition is difficult to diagnose because it's hard to tell whether a person is having normal reactions to stressful circumstances or *over*reactions to stressful circumstances. Dysthymia is a fairly recent label; before 1980, people with these symptoms were simply thought to have a personality/attitude problem, not an illness. Dysthymia may be proof that a person has been exposed to the despair and stresses of life to the extent that he or she can no longer fully enjoy life. Studies show (no surprises here) that people with dysthymia are more likely to develop full-blown, or major, depression; and people with dysthymic relatives are more likely to develop dysthymia. In other words, if your mother had a "difficult" personality, odds are you're not going to be able to cope with life as well—or as calmly—as someone with a mother who had a sunny disposition. Children displaying symptoms of dysthymia (especially if they are growing up in poverty and terrible circumstances) may be diagnosed with early-onset dysthymia.

According to the DSM IV, you may suffer from dysthymic disorder if you've had a depressed mood most days for at least two years but your symptoms are less severe than those suffered from major depression, and you experience two or more of the following:

- Poor appetite or overeating
- Lack of or too much sleep
- Fatigue and low energy

- Low self-image or self-esteem
- Trouble concentrating and making decisions
- Hopelessness about the future

Melancholic Depression

This is similar to major depression, but more severe than a "severe episode" of major depression. If you look at the list of symptoms given on pages 7–8 and add the words *profound*, *extreme*, or *excessive* to each one (as in a "profound loss of energy" and so on), they become the symptoms of melancholic depression.

Double Depression

This is a very confusing term. It refers to the condition of a person who has probably been mildly depressed for some time and is suddenly in the throes of a severe episode of major depression.

Agitated Depression

This is when you're anxious and depressed all at once. You have many of the symptoms of major depression, but you have the added symptoms of anxiety disorders, such as not being able to sit still, feeling restless, and so on.

Psychotic Depression

This is depression with psychotic features. You're depressed *and* you've lost touch with reality. This is quite a bad combination and is characterized by visual hallucinations, hearing voices, having delusions (false beliefs), extreme feelings of worthlessness, and so on. This is frequently misdiagnosed as schizophrenia, and the suicide risk is extremely high in this kind of illness.

10. Understand Treatment Options for Depression

Depression can be treated with short-term or long-term strategies. All of the lifestyle and wellness tips in this book represent long-term approaches for preventing first or recurring episodes of depression without the use of antidepressants. But it's important to know what treatment strategies are currently used for people in the throes of a depression.

Short-Term Strategies

There is no one way to stop the suffering in depression. Different things work for different people. Less invasive solutions involve finding someone to talk to. This translates into finding counseling or psychotherapy. Talk therapy may work best in combination with antidepressants (which this book does not discuss) or self-care strategies (Part V).

Although this book is called *50 Ways to Fight Depression Without Drugs*, it's important to point out that medication may have a role in more serious cases of depression. Consider this analogy. Imagine that you've been pulled from a burning building. If you're wheezing and coughing from smoke inhalation, there's nothing wrong with being prescribed medication that will help you breathe in the short term. But you may also need to talk to somebody about the fire, or talk to other people who have been in a fire. Depression is no different. Medication can help you breathe or stop suffering in the short term, but it can't give you insights for the long term or provide the emotional support you need to see what you need to see, learn what you need to learn, and face what you need to grow through.

Long-Term Strategies

Preventing a recurrence of a depressive episode involves prolonged therapy, including long-term counseling and/or psychotherapy; long-term talk therapy in combination with medications or herbs; and lifestyle changes ranging from stress reduction techniques to dramatic changes involving residence, jobs, and interpersonal relationships. Since these strategies often mean making dramatic changes in your life, which can take a long time to come to terms with or implement, counseling is often a key component in managing depression.

The "sharing" approach used in support groups has been shown to be highly beneficial—particularly in cases where people share difficult circumstances or have difficulties in common.

PART II

Rediscover Passion

11. Know the True Meaning of Passion

When there is an absence of passion, our lives become flat and featureless, a condition otherwise known as depression. Again, this is not characterized so much by sadness as by a numbness or lack of engagement in life. Depression is accompanied by a loss of interest and pleasure in once-enjoyable activities. So, another million-dollar question must be answered: what is passion?

We identify passion with happiness, joy, and sexual fulfillment. It's been equated with sexual intensity, which may be a feature of passion, but in no way defines it. The word *passion* has lost its true meaning for those who feel a sense of monotony in their culture. Ironically, the word itself comes from the root *passio*, which means "suffering." How is it that passion arises from suffering? Researching this concept takes us into an exploration of end-of-life, death-and-dying issues. Without an exploration of such issues, we cannot understand passion.

When we are faced with the death of a loved one or even our own death, the essence of life bubbles forth: real feelings, real suffering, and raw emotions come out. We live on the "edge," waiting for the unknown and calling on all our inner reserves and strength to get through the experience. Death experiences remind us of the precariousness of life and how planning for the future cannot replace living in the present. "Feeling your life" is how I define passion. And nothing is more passionate than dying or being with someone who is dying.

The events of September 11, 2001, show us how tragedy and suffering can crystallize what is truly important to us. Prior to that date, most North Americans never talked about death or even thought about it. We were too busy trying to live longer, look younger, and find miracle cures for disease. The character Morrie in Mitch Albom's *Tuesdays with Morrie* says: "When you know how to die, you know how to live." Death brings us closer to our lives.

12. Feel Your Mortality

When we feel our mortality, we "feel our lives." As we age, we become particularly aware of our mortality—especially when someone our own age is dying. But there are other "markers" of our mortality that may bring us closer to our deaths, and therefore our feelings and our lives. For example, many people "feel" their age on birthdays ending in five or zero; when their youngest child marks an occasion of adulthood, such as graduation, moving out, or marriage; when they watch their parents age, become feeble or disabled; or when they realize they are no longer perceived as young by others (for example, not being noticed by the opposite sex anymore comes as a hard shock for both men and women).

When we experience illness and/or physical vulnerability, life takes on a new meaning and we begin to look at it differently. Gail Sheehy refers to this as the "task of reflection." It is often on making this reflection (have we lived well, are we happy, were we good people, are there things we still want or need to do, etc.), that we become more passionate, but this usually happens when we make a conscious shift to another stage of life. Entering middle age, for example, our health suddenly becomes very important to us; many people become active for the first time or dramatically change their habits—eating well, quitting smoking, and so on.

The deaths of others also affects us differently as we age because it mirrors our progression toward this inevitable event. In fact, Sheehy defines the word *progress* as a series of little victories over little deaths.

Feeling our mortality may sound ominous, but if you didn't know you were going to die one day, you wouldn't find enjoyment in anything you did. There would be no "last piece of cake," sense of time, or feeling of something being over. There would be no meaningful sex either, because the sexual experience is a microcosm of the stages of life, ending in what the French call *le petit mort* or "little death"—their term for orgasm. Nor would there be that last night on a vacation. Without these small, daily reminders that we will not last forever, our lives would be devoid of meaning. At the same time, without endings, there would be no beginnings. There would be nothing new, such as a new food to try, new places to explore, and so on. Without a sense of discovery, there would be no value in art or artists, since it is the uniqueness and newness of an artist's work that we appreciate.

Unless we feel our death, we cannot feel our life. If we knew we would live forever, we would not be concerned with deadlines, productivity, and so forth. In fact, people face their mortality when they make all sorts of decisions that seem to have nothing to do with death on the surface. These may include:

• Making sacrifices for children. (This choice is driven by the sense that your children are the future, and that by ensuring their happiness, your life will have meaning and purpose after your death.)

- Going back to school or retraining for a different profession. (This choice is driven by a feeling that there are still things to do or learn before you die.)

- Leaving a stagnant relationship or marriage. (This choice is driven by the sense that you only live once.)

- Staying in a less than satisfactory relationship in order to have a child or family. (This choice is driven by the need to leave your genetic mark on the world.)

13. Understand Why We Appreciate Beauty

For the most part, beauty does not last, which is why we appreciate it as much as we do. When Diana, former Princess of Wales, was killed in a car crash in 1997, the world went into a state of shock. People from all over the globe felt compelled to travel to London to leave flowers or a card or just "be there." News coverage was continuous, and some news stations called upon psychologists and clergy to help explain why there was such a profound sense of loss over her death. I, too, mourned her death and would inexplicably burst into tears each time I heard Elton John's ode to her on the radio. I was not a royal watcher and was at a loss to explain my reaction. When Mother Teresa died a week later, the Western world was not as moved by her death. Intellectually, we knew that this woman's deeds and the life she had led far outweighed Diana's contributions. Yet we did not mourn for her loss in the same way. Why?

The answer is not complicated: When something beautiful—such as a young, promising life—ends, or ends too soon, we profoundly appreciate the meaning of that ending;

it is a reminder of our own vulnerability. We are vulnerable to damage; we can die at any time. In Diana's case, we were upset by both a life interrupted, and a death that was unnecessary. But for reckless driving, she would not have died. It seemed so senseless. Elton John's tribute to Diana symbolized her as a rose. Why are roses or flowers significant to us? Why do we bother with annuals in our gardens? When something beautiful is taken away before we are ready, we experience the loss as tragedy. But it is through tragedy that we find meaning.

Our appreciation of beauty explains myriad activities people are passionate about, such as bird-watching, hiking, enjoying thunderstorms, and finding rooms with a view.

14. Find Ways to Feel Connected

The large body of work that looks at causes of sadness and depression shows us that people suffer most when they are feeling disconnected from the world around them. When we feel plugged into our community and network of friends and colleagues, it brings us increased zest, well-being, and motivation. Connection brings us feelings of greater self-worth, as well as a desire to make more connections. The flip side of wanting to connect with someone is that we can open up too much and become vulnerable. Vulnerability can, of course, let us be taken advantage of. Most people have a few bitter recollections of times their vulnerability and openness allowed less-than-savory characters into their lives. A lot of us may stray into relationships with people who take terrible advantage of our feelings and generosity. The problem with vulnerability is that it cannot ever be a middle-of-the-road proposition; there is simply no way around the risk of being hurt. That is why many of us learn to shut down; then passion is repressed, which can predispose us to depression or numbness.

Cutting ourselves off from other people can also cause loneliness. Loneliness is stressful; solitude is rejuvenating. Loneliness comes from a lack of truly intimate relationships with friends or family members; intimacy, in this case, refers to sharing deep feelings, fears, and so on with someone. This is how we unburden ourselves and relieve stress. Feeling as though you belong somewhere or are a part of a community can alleviate loneliness. Here are steps you can take to create more supportive relationships in your life:

• Find some sort of social group to belong to. Look into gourmet cooking clubs, art classes, and so on. Find an activity that you're really drawn to, and chances are you'll meet like-minded souls with whom you can form quality friendships.

• Have a couple of nice dinner parties each year. It's a way to create more intimate relationships with people who may only be acquaintances or casual friends.

• Get involved in your community. Whether it's a "not in my backyard" lobby or a community street sale, get out and meet your neighbours. Participating in community-based programs, ranging from arts-and-crafts groups to yoga classes, is a way to find emotional support. In fact, community outreach workers use arts and crafts, fitness, and computer classes as tools to attract people within the community who could benefit from such support. What often takes place in these programs is a great deal of talking and sharing during, prior to, and after the activity. These are places where you can make friends; find someone you can talk to; and most importantly, realize that you're not alone.

- Volunteer. Volunteering for causes dear to your heart is a great way to meet people and feel needed. Meals on Wheels, elder care facilities, street youth programs, and so forth all attract wonderful people with whom you may share friendship and comfort while working to help others. Plus, when you're involved in someone else's life, your own problems seem smaller.

- Get a dog. Dogs need to be walked, which means you'll meet other people walking their dogs. And dog owners tend to gravitate toward other dog owners. It's a great jumping-off point for meeting people. Aside from that, many studies point to the health benefits of owning any sort of pet, including lower blood pressure and reduced incidence of heart disease.

15. Express Your Anger in Healthy Ways

Anger is one of the most vital expressions of passion, but often people in our culture do not feel they are allowed to express it openly. Many turn it on themselves, and it manifests as depression. Or the anger may become misdirected and confused, spawning all kinds of negative behaviors and relationships.

Common manifestations of unexpressed anger include:

- *Depression.* Depression is commonly understood as "anger turned inward." Anger is mobilizing; depression is immobilizing.

- *Eating disorders.* Men tend to overeat; women tend to either binge and purge or starve themselves.

- *Self-harm.* This is a broad category that includes harmful addictions, harmful relationships, suicide attempts, self-mutilation, and self-destructive or self-sabotaging behaviors.

- *Harm to others.* This includes petty crimes, such as theft; vexatious lies (lies that deliberately hurt versus "white lies"); harassment (stalking, repeated phone calls or E-mails); violence; and heinous crimes (murder, or other types of violence against others).

Many people who play subordinate roles either in the home, workplace, or society believe the following:

- I am weak. If I express my anger, I'll be overpowered.

- I am dependent. If I express my anger, I may disrupt my lifestyle.

- I have no right to feel anger. If I express my anger, I won't be liked or loved as much.

- I want people to think I'm nice.

A good behavioral counselor or therapist can help you learn to express anger in healthy ways. This means stating your disappointment at appropriate times rather than holding back and exploding inappropriately at the wrong person. See Part V for more information on finding good counseling.

16. Express Your Creativity

Self-expression is a passionate act. When people put their passion into their work, art (in all its forms—words, fine arts, visual arts, healing arts, performing arts, etc.), hobbies, or sports, they not only feel their lives but express their lives. Creativity is an amazing defense against depression. In particular, writing in the form of journaling, composing poetry, or writing letters is a great way to express yourself and improve your mental health. A new study published in the *Journal of the American Medical Association* found that people suffering from chronic ailments such as asthma or arthritis actually felt better when they wrote about their ailments.

A few years ago, Oprah Winfrey used her influence to get her viewers to begin journaling or diary writing daily because of the powerful way it can enable those who are otherwise without voice or expression. Using her own creativity to enable others, she has resold the idea of journaling in an age where few people take the time to sit down and be still with their thoughts. Oprah has taken journaling one step further by encouraging people to begin "gratitude journaling" in which they think about what they are thankful for in their lives and actually write it down. A firm believer in literacy as well, Oprah's influence on the comeback of journals can help many people, who may have been afraid to try to write because of a lack of education, to find the courage to express themselves in this way. Even if people do not feel they are creative or artistic, journaling is an opportunity for them to express their feelings and passions.

There are other types of creativity as well. Why is Martha Stewart so successful? Because she offers creative rescue for millions through her "lifestyle arts." Martha offers some good suggestions to help change our lifestyles and routines, inviting us to take a different look at life and feel the small things. Whether it's beautiful flowers, crafts, or the hundreds of small things that take hours to make, she offers thousands of creative rescues every day through her television programs, books, magazine, and website.

17. Enjoy Your Food

The French have a saying: Regret nothing in matters of love and food. Puzzled scientists who have been trying to figure out why the French have such low rates of heart disease in spite of their rich diets (known as the French Paradox) have found that the answer is passion. The French are passionate about their food and really enjoy it. They never think of food as sinful; instead, they simply think of it as delicious. To the French, food is a work of art, meant to be enjoyed. To Americans, food is calorie-laden, fattening, and forbidden. They tend to think about food as either fuel or poison; they fear the effect it will have on their bodies. In France, good food feeds the soul, not the body; the French mock the idea of "food police" watching every gram of fat.

They also mock the way Americans eat: Everywhere and anywhere is a dining room. We eat in our cars, walking on the street, and at our desks while we work. In France, eating takes place only in restaurants or at dinner tables at home. The typical American pattern of eating is considered nomadic eating or vagabond feeding and grazing.

There is a huge distinction between the two countries in quantity and quality of food. In the United States, we are taught that large portions are good—even if the food is mediocre or of poor quality. In France, the taste and quality of the food is the most important factor; when the taste is good and the quality of the food is high, the appetite is satiated, making the quantity or portion size unimportant.

When food is enjoyed, endorphins are secreted that help us feel better and relieve stress. One of the most well-known comfort foods, chocolate, has been found to have this effect. And by the way, when you sit down to eat, please use the good dishes! What are you saving them for?

18. Get into a Cause

Causes can be wonderful ways to use your skills, talents, and energies. The number of people who throw themselves into volunteer work is staggering. It amounts to millions of hours. These causes are creative rescues and are one reason why people become possessive about their responsibilities within such organizations.

For instance, in my own experience with nonprofit health organizations, I have encountered hundreds of people who tirelessly devote their bodies and souls to "the cause." But when you ask them about their personal lives, they usually have very mundane, passionless existences. It's a pattern I've come to recognize. Some of the most devoted people do not even have the disease they are raising funds for, nor do they know anyone with that disease. The term *professional volunteer* describes the incredible, energetic, tireless fundraiser who can talk anyone into giving his or her organization a buck. I've seen these people in action, and I am amazed at their passion and dedication.

Causes range from saving elephants from poachers to finding cures for rare diseases most of us have never even heard of. People may become heavily involved in political and environmental causes as a means of creative rescue, giving them a place to use their talents and knowledge. Such causes also offer other fringe benefits, such as travel, if the organization is national and has an annual general meeting. If you're feeling blah with the routine of the everyday, find something that interests you and volunteer. Help the homeless; read to the blind; work in a food bank or soup kitchen. You'll meet nice people who are like-minded, and you'll wind up contributing to someone else's well-being, which will make you feel useful and alive.

19. Do What You Loved as a Child

Children are naturally filled with passion; they're so enamored with life, they don't want to sleep and can barely wait to start each day. Believe it or not, you were like that once, too. Make a list of activities, foods, or places you enjoyed as a child and reenact the memories today. Take a ride on a roller-coaster; have some candy; finger paint; play in the snow; eat dinner backward with dessert first; play with some toys. One passion expert refers to this as "Rekindle-garten." The feelings we had when we did these kinds of things years ago can be brought back, and those feelings can jump-start a childlike quality that can help us feel young and passionate.

That childlike quality has a lot to do with fearlessness. When we try something new, we re-create the wonder we had as children when we tried something for the first time. There are lots of things all of us can try for the first time! Here are a few suggestions:

- Eat at a new restaurant.

- Take in a tourist attraction in your own city that you've never visited.

- Go to a sports event you've never attended before.

- Take an architectural tour of your city, and look at buildings and shapes in a new way.
- Throw a party on the spur of the moment.
- Take dancing lessons.
- Go on a nature adventure (for example, white-water rafting).
- Dress up in formal wear and go to the beach.
- Go for a helicopter ride.

You get the idea! The point is to try something totally new and unlike your daily routine.

20. Talk to Some Passionate People

We all know people who have passion or seem full of life. But when you talk to them, you'll be surprised at how much tragedy and suffering many of them have endured. Passionate people feel their lives by surviving, reinventing themselves, and not being afraid of living. That means not being afraid to sample life and make a few mistakes along the way.

One passion mentor I interviewed refers to life as a sandbox. We can't just sit in the sandbox and not play with the sand; we have to play with it and get a little dirty at times. Another mentor referred to life as a diving board and said that we just have to get in that water regardless of whether it's freezing or muddy or rocky. I'm told by passionate people that life ought to be an emotional adventure. It is the freedom to fail that liberates us most. Says one woman: "Everything we do is training and preparation for something else."

So if you're reflecting on your life and thinking only about the mistakes you've made or your regrets, remember that's what life is for. We're here to try things on and check things out—to feel our bodies and mortality. Einstein said that the person who's never made a mistake has never lived. So, embrace your choices and understand them. You can choose something else tomorrow. Above all, don't be afraid to live. This is your best defense against depression and the best way to truly become yourself. As one person told me: "The older we become, the more ourselves we become."

PART III

Reduce Stress

21. Understand the Meaning of Stress

Generally, stress is defined as a negative emotional experience associated with biological changes that allow you to adapt to it. When you're confronted with a stressful situation, your adrenal glands pump out stress hormones that speed up your body, your heart rate increases, and your blood sugar rises so glucose can be diverted to your muscles in case you have to "run." This is known as the fight or flight response. The hormones produced are called catecholamines, which are broken down into epinephrine (adrenaline) and norepinephrine.

The problem is that the fight or flight response isn't usually necessary in the twenty-first century, because most of our stress stems from interpersonal situations rather than being chased by a predator. Occasionally, we may want to flee from a bank robber or mugger, but most of us just want to flee from our jobs or our kids! In other words, stress hormones actually put a physical strain on our bodies and can lower our resistance to disease. Initially, these hormones stimulate the immune system, but after the original event has passed, they can suppress the immune system, leaving us open to a wide variety of illnesses and all kinds of physical symptoms.

Hans Selye, considered the father of stress management, defined stress as "wear and tear" on the body. Once we are in a state of stress, the body adapts by depleting its resources until it becomes exhausted. The wear and tear on our bodies mounts; we can suffer from any number of stress-related conditions:

• Allergies and asthma
• Back pain

- Cardiovascular problems
- Dental and periodontal problems
- Depression
- Emotional outbursts (rage, crying, irritation)
- Fatigue
- Gastrointestinal problems (digestive disorders and so on)
- Headaches
- Herpes recurrences (especially in women)
- High blood pressure
- High cholesterol
- Immune suppression (predisposing us to viruses, such as colds and flu; infections; autoimmune disorders; and cancer)
- Insomnia
- Loss of appetite and weight loss
- Muscular aches and pains
- Premature aging
- Sexual problems
- Skin problems and rashes

As you can see from this lengthy list, stress greatly contributes to poor health and disease. Addictions and substance abuse may compound many of these problems when we try to relieve our symptoms through recreational substance use or self-medication. Current statistics reveal that 43 percent of all adults suffer from health problems directly caused by stress, while 75 to 90 percent of all visits to primary care physicians are for stress-related complaints or disorders. In the workplace alone, about a million people per day call in sick because of stress, which translates to about 550 million absences per year. Other studies show that roughly 50 percent of all U.S. workers suffer from burnout—a state of mental exhaustion and fatigue caused by stress; 40 percent of employee turnover is directly linked to stress.

Thus, the financial toll of occupational stress to U.S. industry adds up to about $300 billion annually; this figure was arrived at by factoring in absenteeism, lower productivity, employee turnover, and direct medical/legal/insurance fees. California employers spend about $1 billion for medical and legal fees related to worker stress; 90 percent of job-stress lawsuits are successful, paying out four times that of other injury claims. Meanwhile, stress management programs grew from $9.4 billion in 1995 to $11.31 billion in 1999. A more subtle but compelling fact is that in 1997 the word *karoshi*, which means "sudden death from overwork" in Japanese, turned up in English dictionaries.

But worse, terrible industry accidents such as oil spills or nuclear reactor accidents are considered to be caused— 60 to 80 percent of the time—by overstressed workers. Terms such as *office rage*, or *desk rage*, are emerging, too, as workplace violence prompted by stress escalates.

22. Understand the Types of Stress

Managing your stress is no easy feat, particularly since there are different types of stress: acute stress and chronic stress. Acute stress results from an immediate situation, such as organizing a wedding, planning for a conference, or having a blowout on the highway. But there is an end to this stress; when the event passes, so does the stress. There are numerous symptoms of acute stress: anger or irritability, anxiety, depression, tension headaches or migraines, back pain, jaw pain, muscular tension, digestive problems, cardiovascular problems, and dizziness.

But acute stress can be episodic, meaning that one stressful event after another creates a continuous flow of acute stress. Someone who is always taking on too many projects at once is someone who suffers from episodic acute stress. Workaholics and those with so-called Type A personalities are classic sufferers of this type of stress.

I sometimes like to refer to acute stress as "good stress," because good things often come from it, even though it feels bad in the short term. This is the kind of stress that challenges us to stretch ourselves beyond our capabilities, makes us meet deadlines, and encourages us to push the envelope and invent creative solutions to our problems. Examples of good stress include ambitious projects; positive life events (moving, changing jobs, or ending unhealthy relationships); confronting fears, illness, or people who make us feel bad (this is one of those bad-in-the-short-term/good-in-the-long-term situations). Essentially, whenever a stressful event triggers emotional, intellectual, or spiritual growth, it is good stress. It is often not the event as much as it is your response to the event that determines whether stress is good or bad. The death of a loved one can sometimes lead to personal growth because we may discover something about ourselves we did not see before—the ability to be resilient, for example. So even a death can create good stress even though we grieve and are sad for a while.

What I call bad stress is also known as chronic stress. This stems from boredom and stagnation, as well as prolonged negative circumstances. Essentially, when no growth occurs from a stressful event, you have bad stress. When negative events don't seem to yield anything positive in the long term, simply more of the same, the resulting stress can lead to chronic and debilitating health problems. This is not to say that we can't get sick from good stress, too, but when nothing positive comes from stress, it has a much more serious effect on our health. Some examples of bad stress include unfulfilling jobs or relationships, disability from a terrible accident or disease, long-term unemployment, chronic poverty, racism, sexism, age discrimination, religious intolerance, or lack of opportunities for change. These kind of situations can lead to depression, low self-esteem, and a host of physical illnesses.

In addition to acute and chronic stress, stress can be categorized in even more precise ways:

- Physical stress (physical exertion)
- Chemical stress (when we're exposed to toxins in the environment, including drugs and alcohol)
- Mental stress (when we take on too much responsibility and begin worrying about all that has to be done)
- Emotional stress (when feelings such as anger, fear, frustration, sadness, betrayal, and bereavement stress us out)
- Nutritional stress (when we're deficient in certain vitamins or nutrients, have overindulged in fat or protein, or suffer from food allergies)
- Traumatic stress (when we experience trauma to the body such as infection, injury, burns, surgery, or extreme temperatures)

- Psychospiritual stress (when there is unrest in our personal relationships or belief system, personal life goals, and so on; in general, defining whether we are happy)

The bottom line is: *Stress makes us sick.*

23. Recognize Your Job Stress

You may not be aware of how much stress you endure by simply working within the old nine-to-five structure (which is more like five-to-nine for most of us) that still exists in most offices. The workplace is a volatile stress factory for most employees because there is the constant threat of losing your job. Mergers and downsizing have increased job stress for millions. Factor in new bosses, computer surveillance, fewer health and retirement benefits, and the unspoken pressure of "face time" (meaning that you feel the need to hang around the office longer to look like you're productive and dedicated, even though no one has actually told you to stay) and the stress can really affect your personal life.

One of the most significant factors in job stress is a sense of powerlessness over your own job. Secretaries, waitresses, mid-level managers, police officers, editors, and medical interns are considered to have high-stress positions for these reasons. These are jobs with a lot of responsibility but little authority. Poets in desk jobs (highly creative people performing unchallenging jobs to pay the rent) are also thought to be highly stressed. For example, are you an actor by night and a bookkeeper or receptionist by day?

A number of studies note that when you don't control decision-making related to your duties, you endure more chronic stress. Although acute stress often comes with the

responsibility of making decisions, people are more motivated and creatively challenged when they feel their opin-
ions or decisions are valued.

There are also jobs that cause trauma. Criminal justice
personnel, firefighters, ambulance drivers, military personnel, and disaster teams witness horrific scenes each day.
There are also physicians, caregivers, social workers, and
therapists who experience vicarious traumatization, meaning they are adversely affected by what they see and hear
all the time. Even ordinary jobs can be traumatic when
clients threaten you emotionally or physically.

The workplace itself can be stressful to your body if it is
hazardous or toxic in some way. In 1995, Dr. Peter Inante,
Director of the Office of Standards Review, Occupational
Safety and Health Administration of the U.S. Department
of Labor, stated that blue-collar workers "appeared to be
the canaries in our society for identifying human chemical
carcinogens in the general environment." Known carcinogens in the office (or home) may be found in:

- Asbestos building materials
- Cleaning products and disinfectants
- Urea-formaldehyde foam insulation
- Adhesives (may contain naphthalene, phenol,
  ethanol, vinyl chloride, formaldehyde, acrylonitrile,
  and epoxy, which are toxic substances that release
  vapors)
- Toners used in copy machines and printers
- Particleboard furniture and space dividers
- Permanent-ink pens and markers (contain acetone,
  cresol, ethanol, phenol, toluene, and xylene)

- Polystyrene cups

- Secondhand smoke

- Synthetic office carpet (may contain acrylic, polyester, and nylon plastic fibers; formaldehyde-based finishes; and pesticides due to mothproofing of wool)

- Correction fluid (may contain cresol, ethanol, trichloroethlyene, and naphthalene, which are all toxic chemicals)

You're more likely to be affected by workplace carcinogens if you:

- work or live in an energy-sealed building;

- are exposed to fumes from carpets, pesticides, cleaners, and airborne allergens

- are exposed to industrial chemicals, such as those found in plants that process wood, metal, plastics, paints, and textiles;

- are in constant contact with pesticides, fungicides, and fertilizers;

- live in a high-pollution area; and/or

- work in dry cleaning, hair styling, pest control, or printing and photocopying.

For more information, you can go to the National Institute of Occupational Safety and Health (NIOSH) website at: cdc.gov/niosh.

NIOSH Information Dissemination can also be accessed directly by calling (513) 533-8287. You can also consult the Centers for Disease Control and Prevention (CDC) in Atlanta at (404) 639-3311. Finally, you can contact the

Occupational Safety and Health Administration (OSHA) by visiting osha.gov. OSHA is the federal agency in charge of worker safety and health.

24. Try to Do What You Love

If you do what you love, you'll love what you do. And you'll feel a lot better, even though you may not make as much money. Surveys and studies show across the board that stress is created by going to a job you hate every day. Doing what you love doesn't mean throwing in the towel and moving to France so you can paint for the rest of your life. It means exploring what you're good at and/or enjoy doing to see whether there's a way you can earn an income from it. For example, does anyone offer adult courses you can take that would allow you to enter a field you prefer? The promise of a more enjoyable job/career with the right credentials often reduces chronic stress. So, although expanding your education or training may involve some short-term stress vis-à-vis added responsibilities, it gives you more hope for the future, which reduces stress in the long run.

Sometimes doing what you love means facing the fact that you're not very good at directing others and would prefer a nonmanagerial position. Working in the store instead of running it is often the solution, which can be arranged within your company. On the flip side, doing what you love might mean realizing that you *are* a leader and find it stressful to be in a subordinate position. In this case, starting your own company, where you have control, may be less stressful for you, even though it involves far more responsibility. This is one reason why Internet businesses are exploding; these home-based businesses, many founded by women, are becoming much easier to start in light of new technologies and the instant availability of the global marketplace. Moving to a position in a large company that allows you to be an intrapreneur, someone who develops new enterprises within a corporation, can be a very satisfying solution when you crave more control or leadership responsibilities.

Or maybe you want to avoid an office environment altogether. There are millions of traveling salespeople who are supplied with gas or car allowances and work mostly on commission with a small base salary. For many, these positions offer the flexibility and lifestyle control that enables them to feel autonomous.

Some people reduce job stress by taking a simple side job with flexible hours to allow them time to pursue their art or main interest. Couriers, postal workers, restaurant servers, and others frequently have more artistic lifestyles after work. When the job simply supports their passion rather than consuming their lives, it becomes far less stressful because its importance is diminished. Lose one side job and it's easy to get another; in other words, side jobs allow for detachment, whereas career jobs involve attachment and far more emotional investment.

Sometimes you need to face up to the fact that your dream job or profession has become a living nightmare. This is not an easy thing to admit, but everyone has a breaking point. For instance, it's the point at which the overworked medical resident in a busy university teaching hospital, who spends most of her time filling out insurance paperwork, decides that she's packing up and becoming a general practitioner in an underserviced rural area. So, she won't become the brilliant heart surgeon her family dreamed of; so, she won't earn $350,000 per year. Instead, she'll settle for a third of that salary in a peaceful country setting where the housing is affordable, people say hello to her, and she can focus on caring for patients.

Pursuing what you love involves these steps:

1. Ask yourself whether you're happy with your choice of job or career. Being happy is not the same thing as feeling stable or "not miserable." If you're not happy, persistently working in a state of unhappiness is unhealthy.

2. Make a list of dream jobs or careers — no matter how silly you think they sound. Did you always want to be a dancer but ended up making a living in marketing? Maybe you can pursue administrative or marketing jobs with a dance company or theatre. Maybe you can write about dance or start a children's dance school. Have you always wanted to be a farmer? Why not? Organic farming is booming! Dream jobs can also mean parenting. If being a stay-at-home parent is your dream, it's worth pursuing.

3. Decide whether you hate your profession — or just your job or locale. How portable is your profession? If you can take it anywhere — for example, you're a webmaster, writer, or teacher — find a more suitable city or town to live in and just start working. Many careers can be turned into home-based businesses through the Internet. Are you a burnt-out secretary? Start your own secretarial service on the Web. (If there isn't a secretary.com yet, someone ought to start one!)

4. Talk to family members and see whether they'll support you in pursuing something else. If they're not behind you, doing what you love may be more difficult — and may make you face deeper questions about your emotional sup-

port system. Sometimes it's necessary to leave relationships or marriages when it comes to going after your dreams. In assessing what you want, you may find that you've been simply going through the motions all these years and need a more equitable, nurturing relationship.

25. Reduce the Commute

One of the simplest ways to de-stress is to eliminate that lengthy commute. If you live in a suburban community and drive into an urban center, you may be spending more than an hour each way, to and from work. This kind of driving is stressful, and reducing your time behind the wheel can reduce a lot of anxiety. Here are some ways to shorten your commute:

• If you spend most of your time at work on a computer or the phone, try to negotiate with your employer for telecommuting. This means plugging into the workplace from home. With teleconferencing tools, there's often little reason to actually go into an office these days. Your employer can save on overhead because of the office space you'll free up and may attract more loyal employees by giving them more flexibility. (And remind your boss that telecommuters do not spend their days at home watching TV!)

• Look into moving closer to work. If you calculate your expenses for car maintenance, gas, and so on, moving within walking distance of your office may be the answer. A lot of people find trading their house in the suburbs for a rental in the city makes more sense financially. Rent and no car often equals far less than a mortgage and two cars!

Car rentals for weekends away and the occasional taxi still add up to less money than car lease fees, financing payments, repairs, gas, and insurance.

• If there's no way you can move, no way your employer will let you work from home, and you're working very late hours anyway, consider renting a small apartment or room within walking distance of your office. Leave the car at the office weekdays and crash in your small "city space." Drive home on weekends. Of course, if this creates more stress because of problems at home, don't do it, but a lot of commuters are finding a small city crash pad has other advantages. You can extend its use to visiting friends or relatives (remember, though, that hosting visitors often creates more stress!), and other family members can stay there when they have to be in the city for extended periods of time. Sometimes marriages and long-term relationships even benefit when there's a place for one partner to go for personal space or distance in high-stress times.

26. Make Less Time for Work

Cutting down from a five-day work week to a four-day work week greatly reduces stress for many people. Psychologically, working Tuesday to Friday eliminates Monday. According to Deepak Chopra, more people have heart attacks on Monday morning than at any other time. Monday to Thursday is another popular choice, giving you an early start to your weekend. If you're a valued employee, many companies would rather have you working for them four days a week than not at all. When you calculate the time it takes to train someone else, it's more costly to replace you than to give you your shorter week. You simply reduce your salary to accommodate your new schedule.

Other ways to negotiate a reduced work week include using vacation and sick days as Mondays off for a year. Some executives have weeks of vacation time they've never taken that can be used to shorten the week. In some companies, being away from the office for long periods of time actually creates more stress and guilt for the employee, so taking a day off each week may be a solution to "vacation-itis." Another way to cut down your time at work is to see whether someone else in the office wants to job share. Surveys show that most people would trade in full-time hours for part-time if they could have job security. The *Miami Herald* proved the point by allowing two very stressed-out female reporters to share their jobs. The result was that the two less stressed and very happy women produced the best work of all the reporters!

You Need a Vacation!

A study done by the American Psychosomatic Society on 12,338 men, aged thirty-five to fifty-seven, found that those who took annual vacations were 21 percent less likely to die during the sixteen-year study period than nonvacationers—and 32 percent less likely to die of coronary heart disease. This is not at all surprising. Two weeks is not enough vacation time for the average person. European companies routinely offer six weeks of vacation. When you renegotiate your vacation package, offer to combine paid vacation with unpaid leave. Surveys show that most people would gladly take unpaid vacation time if they were guaranteed job security.

A more dramatic move is to look into taking a sabbatical. This means taking a year off without pay for family reasons (stress reduction, mental health, etc.). Again, many people would take the time off if they could be guaranteed job security upon their return. Sabbatical leave is offered to some professionals, such as teachers and tenured professors at universities, but there's no reason why it shouldn't be an option for other workers. Cashing in some retirement funds to finance your year away from work could pay off in the form of physical, mental, and emotional rejuvenation.

27. Rid Yourself of E-Stress

For most of us, E-mail, voice mail, cell phones, pagers, and all the technology that is part of everyday life have only lengthened our workdays and given us less time to ourselves. Twenty-five years ago, when you called someone who wasn't home, the phone rang a lot and that was it. There was no onus on the "other person" to return your call; it was your responsibility to call back if you needed to get in touch. But with voice mail and answering machines, the burden is on the person receiving the call to return it—and even to answer numerous calls simultaneously with the advent of call waiting.

Today, even more technology—in the form of call screening—is required to avoid phone calls. The greater access to communication that technology provides makes our "to do" lists much longer. And if you've made the mistake of subscribing to Internet server lists, known as listservs, you could become bombarded with E-mails, as many as hundreds per day. The benefits and burdens of technology increase with Palm Pilots, laptops, and so forth. Even watching television has become infinitely more complicated with complex remotes that power the VCR, stereo system, and digital cable box as well.

All this translates to E-stress, part of which is caused by the learning curve. Learning how to use each new technological toy can wreak havoc on the central nervous system. And it seems the learning never ends, as new gadgets are introduced every few months that make the old gadget obsolete. New versions of E-mail or fax software also cause ongoing problems.

Another part of E-stress is the lack of privacy. With so many ways for people to contact us, there is no safe haven that is communication-free. With each new mode of communication comes more responsibility to reply. Experts call this multitasking madness. And who hasn't been forced to listen to the details of someone else's private life in a public place owing to an overly loud cell-phone conversation? We've all had those moments where we've glared at someone because we really didn't need to know about their mother's friend's colonoscopy.

All the E-stuff in your life interferes with normal communication. When you're E-mailing with one hand, holding the phone with the other, and hearing your pager go off at the same time, how much attention can you give any of these interactions? The first step in turning down the "E" is looking at all the ways you're plugged in each day. Answer these questions:

• How many phone lines do you have?

• How do you receive the Internet? If it's via cable or dedicated line, you're never "off."

• How many ways can people reach you?

• How many messages do you receive through each of these modes? Count everything: E-mail to your office, E-mail to your home, messages to your cell phone and office voice mail, calls to your answering machine at home, and so on.

• Does E-mail enhance your interpersonal relationships or detract from them? For example, do you find yourself feeling isolated in spite of all the ways you can contact people? Does your life partner spend his or her time at home with you or with his or her computer? Do you share quality time with your children, or do they spend all of their time at home online or playing video and computer games? A 2000 Stanford University study on the societal impact of the Internet found that Internet use caused social isolation, which confirmed the findings of a 1998 study by researchers at Carnegie Mellon University.

Reducing E-stress involves redesigning the technology in your life to work for you rather than against you. Implementing just one of the following steps can help:

• Set up unplugged time. Make a decision to shut down by a certain time each day, such as after six in the evening and on weekends. You can even indicate your unplugged zone on your outgoing voice-mail message: "Hi. You've reached Dale at 555-5555. I check my voice mail between nine and six each day. After that time, I cannot be reached." Turn off your computer after six, too, and do not check E-mail with your cell phone or Palm Pilot beyond that time. You can set up automatic E-mail responses that tell people you're away, busy, not answering, and so on.

• Use your cell phone only in case of an emergency. Don't give out the number to anyone other than immediate family members, and don't turn it on unless you absolutely have to. If you have voice mail and E-mail, people don't really need to reach you by cell phone. Don't subscribe to a message service on your cell phone either. That way, no one can leave messages.

• Limit your gadgets. If you've survived this long without a Palm Pilot, do you really need one? The more stuff you buy, the more you'll use and the less time you'll have.

• Limit your surfing time. If you're searching for information about a topic on the Internet (such as stress), you could be there for days. Give yourself a limited amount of time for research and say (as I do), "I've done the best I can with the time I have."

• Limit the number of messages you save. Try to write down information as you get it and erase the message. Otherwise, you'll spend too much time listening to old messages.

• Eliminate phone tag by leaving a specific message with specific instructions for replying: "Hi, George. This is Su Lin. I wanted to set up a meeting this Thursday, at 1:00 P.M., in front of the Coffee Mill. If you can't make it, E-mail me with an alternate time and place. Otherwise, I'll see you Thursday."

28. Eliminate Energy Drains

Most energy drains are people. When you're surrounded by people who take energy from you rather than give it to you in the form of support, the result is more stress. By doing a serious reevaluation of your personal relationships, you may be able to find more energy and reduce the amount of stress in your life. Ask yourself some of the following questions:

• Do you have someone in your life who offers emotional support without judgment? This means a person who makes you feel positive about yourself and doesn't point out your flaws or attack your choices.

• Are there people in your life who drain your energy and reserves? These are people who always seem to be having a crisis and suck up large amounts of free therapy time from you, but are never there when you need them. They can also be people who criticize you and make you feel negative and hopeless instead of positive and optimistic.

• Do you have unresolved conflicts with family members or friends? Such feelings can drain your energy and focus because you tend to obsess over the conflict again and again (see Part V).

• Do you feel your friends are more like acquaintances and you lack truly intimate friendships?

• Do you feel a void in your life because you have no romantic partner?

• Are you in a romantic or sexual relationship that you need to end, but have been avoiding taking the necessary steps?

• Are you in a relationship that compromises your values?

• Is there a phone call you need to make but are avoiding, which is causing you stress and anxiety? For example, are you avoiding apologizing to someone, or on the flip side, confronting someone? Are you putting off calls to local nursing homes for your aged mother?

• Is there someone in your life who continually breaks commitments or plans and with whom you are constantly rescheduling?

Energy drains also result from unmet needs in your home environment. Do you have broken appliances, car repairs that haven't been done, a wardrobe you hate, cluttered closets and rooms, or even ugly surroundings? Living in a home that is not decorated in a way that pleases you makes you feel you don't want to be there. Plants, paint, covers for ugly furniture, and a few pictures on the walls often make the difference between barren and cozy. See Part V for more on the little things in life that can make a huge difference in your stress quotient.

Finally, energy drains come from procrastinating and overbooking yourself. We often procrastinate over things we really don't want to do—such as taxes. We overbook ourselves when we're afraid of saying no. Every article and book on stress management has those trite three words of advice: Just say no. The problem is that few people ever say it. Instead of "no," try "Let me check my schedule and see whether I'm free." Then, "Sorry, looks like I'm committed elsewhere" or if it's a specific task, "I've got a deadline on that date for something of equal importance."

Finally, simply doing too much and expecting too much from yourself drains your energy. When possible, hire someone to do the things you can't or don't want to do. When you're overworked at the office, subcontracting one or two projects to a freelancer may be an ideal solution. If you don't think your employer will pay for a freelancer, consider sending out the dreaded task on the sly and paying for it out of your own pocket. The job security, perceived good performance, and weight off your shoulders may be worth a couple of hundred bucks. At home, think about hiring someone to do the drudge work you dread:

- Cleaning your house or apartment
- Decluttering rooms by going through closets, filing things, and so on
- Organizing your tax receipts
- Gardening and/or taking care of your lawn

29. Reduce Your Snail Mail and Plastic

Mail is stressful. Do you have what I call "the dining room table problem"? Your mail gets sorted and piled on the dining room table night after night, to the point where the surface of the table disappears and you can never have company because that would mean sorting your mail. If this sounds familiar, you probably have too much unnecessary mail. Calling companies and requesting your name be removed from mailing lists is often just another thing you have to do, so it doesn't get done. The easiest way to reduce the amount of mail that comes in your door is to place a garbage can or recycling bin right by your mailbox so you can sort the mail outside. All flyers and direct mailings (people asking for donations or selling new products, credit cards, or services) go immediately into the garbage. Don't even open them! Postcards, thank-you notes, and so on should be read on the spot, but unless you feel some dire need to save them, toss them out afterward.

The next task is going through your bills and figuring out what can be paid by phone or online. Can you request a stop on snail mail bills and ask for E-mail billings? Can you prepay or prearrange bills to be paid automatically by credit card or debit card and just get notice of monthly payments (such as utilities) on your credit card bill?

As for the plastic, so much mail and stress is generated by credit cards, it's amazing. If you have too many credit cards, you're probably spending more than you can afford and accumulating massive debts. The best credit cards to have are those that give you something in return, such as frequent flyer miles. Pick one card and fly with it! Or pick two—one for personal use and one for business use. Toss all the department store cards (and the various loyalty programs attached to them, which can mean more cards).

Before you cut up the cards you're not going to use anymore, be sure to pay the accounts in full, and tell the credit card company you're closing your account. Some companies require you to return the cut-up plastic.

Finally, try to reduce your newspaper and magazine clutter by subscribing to a few of them online. For example, most major daily papers are now on the Web, or at least the local information you need from them is.

30. Restructure Your Finances

Debt is a big stress producer, and feeling the pressures of saving for retirement can add to the problem. While reducing your plastic is one small way of restructuring your finances, another way is to restructure your life so you're financing as little as possible. Here are some ways to do that:

• Get rid of your mortgage. If your house is mortgaged to the hilt or in need of expensive renovations that you can't afford, that causes anxiety. Many people find selling the "money pit" house and buying or renting something cheaper eliminates a lot of debt and worry.

• Get rid of your car. If you're a two-car family, try living with only one car. If you're a one-car family, getting rid of a car is usually only possible in large urban centers with good public transportation. If you can, try living car-free for a year and see whether it makes a difference to your money situation. Gas, repairs, insurance, tickets, parking, and finance payments really add up.

• Use retirement funds to pay off credit card debts or other nagging debts. Your retirement savings don't have to be used just for retirement. You're saving your money to help yourself in the future. Maybe the time to use some of that money is now. Get rid of those high-interest debts once and for all. The money you save by not paying interest can go back into your retirement account.

• Resist the pressure to play the market. There is a lot of pressure from fund management companies to invest your money in high-risk stocks or money market accounts in exchange for higher interest. You could certainly make money on these ventures, but you can lose it, too. If you can't afford to lose, don't play. Keeping your money in accounts with guaranteed or lower interest that are less volatile may give you peace of mind—something that can be more valuable than a piece of the action! When you consider the time spent checking the market, worrying about fluctuations in prices, and so on, it's a lot of wasted energy. Getting your time back may be more valuable than the stock itself.

PART IV

The Physical, Nutritional, and Herbal Approach

31. Understand What Exercise Really Means

When your body is healthy, your mind is healthier, too, which can dramatically reduce episodes of depression. The Oxford dictionary defines exercise as "the exertion of muscles, limbs, etc., especially for health's sake; bodily, mental or spiritual training." In the West, we have placed an emphasis on bodily training when we talk about exercise, completely ignoring the mental and spiritual aspects. Only recently have Western studies begun to focus on the mental benefits of exercise. (It's been shown, for example, that exercise creates endorphins, hormones that make us feel good.) But we still do not encourage meditation or other calming forms of mental and spiritual practice that improve well-being and health—particularly by reducing stress, a major risk factor for depression.

For thousands of years, exercise in the East has focused on achieving mental and spiritual health *through* the body, as in using breathing and postures. Deep breathing and aerobic exercise increase oxygen flow in the body, and when we have more oxygen, we burn fat, our breathing improves, our blood pressure goes down, and our heart works better. Oxygen also lowers triglycerides and cholesterol, increasing our high-density lipoproteins (HDL), or good cholesterol, and decreasing our low-density lipoproteins (LDL), or bad cholesterol. This means that our arteries may unclog, and we may significantly cut our risk of heart disease and stroke. More oxygen makes our brain work better, so we feel better. Studies show that depression is lessened when the oxygen flow in the body increases. Ancient techniques, such as yoga, that specifically improve mental and spiritual well-being achieve this by combining deep breathing and stretching, which improves both oxygen and blood flow.

Nor should we ignore the benefits of cultural traditions such as traditional dances; active prayers that incorporate physical activity; aboriginal healing circles that involve community and communication; and even sweat lodges, believed to help rid the body of toxins through perspiration. These are all wellness activities you may wish to investigate.

32. Discover Your Life Force

All ancient cultures—whether Native American, Indian, Chinese, Japanese, or ancient Greek or Roman—believed there were two fundamental aspects to the human body: the actual physical shell (clinically called the corporeal body) that made cells, blood, tissue, and so on; and an energy flow that made the physical body come alive. The latter was known as the life force or life energy. In fact, this theory is so central to other cultures' view of human function that each has its own word for life force. In China, it is called *qi* (pronounced "chee"). In India, it's called *prana*; in Japan, *ki*. The ancient Greeks called it *pneuma*, which has become a prefix in medicine having to do with the breath and lungs.

Today, Western medicine concentrates on the corporeal body and usually fails to recognize the life force. However, in traditional (non-Western) healing, it is believed that the life force heals the body, not the other way around!

Most traditional healers look on the parts of the body as windows or maps to the body's health. In China, the ears are a complex map, with each point on the ear representing a different organ and part of the psyche. In reflexology, the feet are "read" to tell us about the rest of the body and the spirit. In Ayurveda, the tongue is examined, while other traditions read the iris of the eyes, and so on. Western medicine doesn't really do this. Instead, it looks at every individual part for symptoms of a disease and treats each part individually.

Let's say you notice blurred vision. You might go to an optometrist who gives you a prescription for glasses and sends you on your way. But if you were to go to a doctor of Chinese medicine, you will be told that the degeneration of your eyes points to an unhealthy liver. To the Chinese, the eyes are a direct window to the liver. (Interestingly, it is the eyes that turn yellow when you're jaundiced.) So, instead of giving you a prescription for glasses, the Chinese healer will look into deeper causes of this liver imbalance. You'll be asked about your personal relationships, your diet, your emotional well-being, and your job. The treatment may involve a host of dietary changes, stress-relieving exercises, and herbal remedies. An Ayurvedic doctor may use your tongue to diagnosis the same liver imbalance, but the approach is the same. You'll be asked about your diet, lifestyle, work habits, and so on. In other words, these practitioners do not see the body as separate from the self. To them, what makes us who we are basically has to do with our individual personalities and our societal roles—who we marry, where we work, and how we feel about those things being just as important as our visual problems.

One of the most ancient forms of healing involves energy healing, which can involve therapeutic, or healing, touch. These techniques are considered forms of biofield therapy. An energy healer will use his or her hands to help guide the energy of your life force. The hands may rest on or just close to the body without actually touching it. Energy healing is used to reduce pain and inflammation, improve sleep patterns and appetite, and reduce stress. Supported by the American Holistic Nurses Association, it has been incorporated into conventional nursing practice with good results. Typically, the healer will move loosely cupped hands in a symmetric fashion over your body, sensing cold, heat, or vibration. The healer's hands are then placed over areas where the life energy is unbalanced in order to restore and regulate the energy flow.

All forms of hands-on healing work in some way with life energy. Therapies that help to move or stimulate this energy include:

- Healing touch
- Huna
- Mari-el
- Qi gong
- Reiki

33. Start Living Actively Instead of Aerobically

The phrase *aerobic activity* means that the activity causes your heart to pump harder and faster and causes you to breathe faster, which increases oxygen flow. Activities such as cross-country skiing, walking, hiking, and biking are all aerobic.

But you know what? Exercise practitioners hate the terms *aerobic activity* or *aerobics program* because they are not about what people do in daily life. Health promoters are replacing these terms with *active living*, because that's what becoming nonsedentary is all about. There are many ways that you can adopt an active lifestyle. Here are some suggestions:

- If you drive everywhere, pick the farthest parking space from your destination so you can integrate some daily walking into your life.
- If you take public transportation everywhere, get off one or two stops early so you can walk the rest of the way.
- Choose to take the stairs over escalators or elevators.
- Park at one side of the mall and then walk to the other.
- Take a stroll around your neighborhood after dinner.
- Volunteer to walk the dog.
- On weekends, go to the zoo or get out to flea markets, garage sales, and so on.

34. Calm Your Nerves with Herbs

A wide variety of "nerve herbs" is available over the counter at most drugstores or health food stores; in fact, U.S. sales of botanical products reached an estimated $4.3 billion in 1998, according to *Nutrition Business Journal*. An herb that is described as nervine has a positive effect on the nervous system. It may be toning, relaxing, stimulating, antidepressive, or analgesic. Many people find the following herbal supplements helpful in combating the range of emotional symptoms stress can create, such as irritability, anxiety, sleeplessness, and mild to moderate depression.

St. John's Wort

Also known as hypericum, this has been used as a sort of nerve tonic in folk medicine for centuries. It's been shown to successfully treat mild to moderate depression and anxiety. Used in Germany for years as a first-line treatment for depression, it is endorsed by the American Psychiatric Association. In Germany and other parts of Europe, it outsells Prozac. Since it was introduced in the United States in the early 1990s, it has been used to treat millions of Americans successfully for depression.

The benefits of St. John's wort are that it has minimal side effects, can be mixed with alcohol, is nonaddictive, and does not require ever-increasing doses as antidepressants do. You can go on and off St. John's wort as you wish without any problem; it helps you sleep and dream; it doesn't have any sedative effect and can actually enhance your alertness.

Kava Root

From the black pepper family, kava (*Piper methysticum*) has been a popular herbal drink in the South Pacific for centuries. It grows on the islands of Polynesia and is known to calm the nerves; it eases stress, fatigue, and anxiety, resulting in an antidepressant effect. Kava can also help to alleviate migraine headaches and menstrual cramps. Placebo-controlled studies conducted by the National Institute of Mental Health showed that kava significantly relieved anxiety and stress, without the problem of dependency or addiction. It should not be combined with alcohol, because it can make the effects of alcohol more potent. You should also check with your doctor before you combine kava with any prescription medications.

Sam-e

Sam-e (say: *Sammy*) stands for S-adenosylmethionine, a natural compound made by your body's cells. This compound helps alleviate anxiety and mild depression. Since it was introduced in the United States in March 1999, more people have purchased Sam-e than St. John's wort. It has been shown to help relieve joint pain and improve liver function as well, which makes it popular with people suffering from arthritis. Studies done in Italy during the 1970s documented Sam-e's effectiveness as an antidepressant; recent U.S. studies confirm these results. Some people have reported hot, itchy ears as a side effect.

Gamma-aminobutyric Acid (GABA)

This amino acid is reportedly an antianxiety agent that may also help you fall asleep if you suffer from insomnia.

Inositol

This naturally occurring antidepressant is present in many foods, such as vegetables, whole grains, milk, and meat, and should be available over the counter.

Dehydroepiandrosterone (DHEA)

This hormone is produced by the adrenal glands; production declines as we age. It has been shown to improve moods and memory in certain studies.

Melatonin

This hormone improves sleep and helps reset the body's natural clock. Many people find that this is a helpful herb to combat "jet lag," but the herb is still unavailable in Canada and other countries because of inconclusive information on side effects. Please consult an herbal practitioner and your doctor about possible side effects.

Phosphatidylserine (PS)

This phospholipid feeds brain-cell membranes. Some studies show it has natural antidepressant qualities.

Tetrahydrobiopterin (BH4)

This substance activates enzymes that control serotonin, noradrenaline, and dopamine levels, which are all important for stable moods. Some studies indicate that BH4 is an effective natural treatment for depression.

Phenylethylamine (PEA)

Small quantities of this nitrogen-containing compound are found in the brain. Studies show it works as a natural antidepressant.

Rubidium

Rubidium is a natural chemical in our bodies and belongs to the same family as lithium, potassium, and sodium. It has worked as an antidepressant in some studies.

Ginkgo

This plant is used to treat a variety of ailments and is a common herb in Chinese medicine. It can improve memory, and some studies show that it can boost the effectiveness of antidepressant medications.

Valerian Root

This is similar to kava root in that it works as an antianxiety agent and combats insomnia. When you brew valerian root with passion flower, oat straw, or chamomile, the resulting tea is very relaxing, toning, and restorative.

Ginseng

This helps you adapt better to stress (both physical and psychological). It is also thought to boost the immune system.

Astragalus

Similar to ginseng, this Chinese herb helps you adapt to stress by strengthening the immune system.

35. Try Flower Power

One of the most popular natural emotional "rescues" people are turning to in droves are what's known as the Bach flower remedies. The Bach flower remedies are thirty-eight homeopathically prepared plant and flower liquid extracts. Each flower remedy is designed to treat a different emotion. Dr. Edward Bach invented this healing tradition in the 1930s (during a time of extreme economic and social misery). Bach classified emotions into seven major groups (for example, fear, uncertainty, or loneliness) and thirty-eight different emotional states, and developed corresponding flower remedies. These remedies work through homeopathic principles, stimulating the body's own capacity to heal itself. The flower remedies are made available as a liquid that is preserved in brandy. Taking the remedy involves diluting two drops of the pure liquid into 30 milliliters of mineral water. You then take four drops of the dilution orally four times a day. You can also put two drops of the pure remedy into a glass of water, and just sip it throughout the day.

A complete list of the Bach flower remedies can be found at bachcentre.com/centre/remedies.htm.

Rescue Remedy

Rescue Remedy is a combination of five Bach flower remedies: Cherry Plum, Clematis, Impatiens, Rock Rose, and Star of Bethlehem. This combination works well for people who suffer from panic attacks or anxiety, and is designed to be taken pure, or "neat," from the bottle. You don't need to buy all of the Bach flower remedies and combine them yourself; Rescue Remedy comes premixed. People can either take four drops of Rescue Remedy at once, orally, or dilute four drops in a glass of water and drink. Rescue Remedy reportedly works very quickly to calm the emotions.

36. Consider Aromatherapy

Essential oils, extracted from plants (mostly herbs and flowers), can do wonders to relieve stress naturally; many are known for their calming and antidepressant effects. The easiest way to use essential oils is in a warm bath; you simply put a few drops of the oil into the water, sit back, and relax in it for about ten minutes. The oils can also be inhaled (place a few drops in a bowl of hot water, lean over the bowl with a towel over your head, and breathe); diffused (use a lamp ring or a ceramic diffuser); or sprayed into the air as a mist. The following essential oils are known to have calming, sedative, and/or antidepressant properties:

- Cedarwood
- Chamomile

- Clary sage
- Geranium
- Jasmine
- Lavender (A few drops on your pillow will also help you sleep.)
- Marjoram
- Neroli
- Orange blossom
- Patchouli
- Rose
- Sage
- Sandalwood
- Ylang-ylang

The following scents are considered stimulating and energizing:

- Grapefruit
- Lemon
- Peppermint
- Pine
- Rosemary

37. Eat Well

We now know that a variety of daily nutrients help to regulate our stress levels and our moods. Tryptophan, for example, which is found in milk and other dairy products, helps our bodies build neurotransmitters such as serotonin.

The B vitamins are also important for mental well-being. Vitamin B_{12} is crucial for good general health, while other B-complex vitamins (thiamine, riboflavin, niacin, pyridoxine, pantothenic acid, and biotin) are essential for brain function, enabling you to be cognizant and alert. Folate (also known as folic acid) is particularly important for a healthy mood. Calcium and magnesium help your brain properly transmit nerve impulses. When you don't have enough of these brain foods, you can become more prone to stress, anxiety, or depression. The following list tells you where to find various nutrients in natural sources:

- *Vitamin A (beta carotene).* Vitamin A is found in liver, fish oils, egg yolks, whole milk, butter; beta carotene in leafy greens, and yellow and orange vegetables and fruits. Depleted by coffee, alcohol, cortisone, mineral oil, fluorescent lights, liver cleansing, excessive intake of iron, and lack of protein.

- *Vitamin B_6.* Found in meats, poultry, fish, nuts, liver, bananas, avocados, grapes, pears, egg yolks, whole grains, and legumes. Depleted by coffee, alcohol, tobacco, sugar, raw oysters, and birth control pills.

- *Vitamin B_{12}.* Found in meats, dairy products, eggs, liver, fish. Depleted by coffee, alcohol, tobacco, sugar, raw oysters, and birth control pills.

- *Vitamin C.* Found in citrus fruits, broccoli, green pepper, strawberries, cabbage, tomatoes, cantaloupe, potatoes, and leafy greens. Herbal/other plant sources include rose hips, yellow dock root, raspberry leaf, red clover, hops, nettles, pine needles, dandelion greens, alfalfa, echinacea, skullcap, parsley, cayenne, and paprika. Depleted by antibiotics, aspirin and other pain relievers, coffee, stress, aging, smoking, baking soda, and high fever.

- *Vitamin D.* Found in fortified milk, butter, leafy green vegetables, egg yolks, fish oils, liver, sunlight, and shrimp. There are no herbal sources. Depleted by mineral oil used on the skin, frequent baths, sunscreens with SPF 8 or higher.

- *Vitamin E.* Found in nuts, seeds, whole grains, fish liver oils, leafy greens, kale, cabbage, and asparagus. Herbal/other plant sources are alfalfa, rose hips, nettles, dong quai, watercress, dandelions, seaweeds, wild seeds. Depleted by mineral oil and sulphates.

- *Vitamin K.* Found in leafy greens, corn and soybean oils, liver, cereals, dairy products, meats, fruits, egg yolks, and blackstrap molasses. Herbal/other plant sources are nettles, alfalfa, kelp, and green tea. Depleted by x-rays, radiation, air pollution, enemas, frozen foods, antibiotics, rancid fats, and aspirin.

- *Thiamine (vitamin B_1).* Found in asparagus, cauliflower, cabbage, kale, spirulina (blue-green algae), seaweed, and citrus fruits. Herbal/other plant sources are peppermint, burdock, sage, yellow dock, alfalfa, red clover, fenugreek, raspberry leaves, nettles, catnip, watercress, yarrow, briar rose buds, and rose hips.

- *Riboflavin (vitamin B_2).* Found in beans, greens, onions, seaweed, spirulina, dairy products, and mushrooms. Herbal/other plant sources are peppermint, alfalfa, parsley, echinacea, yellow dock, hops, dandelion, ginseng, dulse, kelp, and fenugreek.

- *Pyridoxine (vitamin B₆)*. Found in baked potato skin, broccoli, prunes, bananas, dried beans and lentils, all meats, poultry, and fish.

- *Folic acid (B factor)*. Found in liver, eggs, leafy greens, yeast, legumes, whole grains, nuts, fruits (bananas, orange juice, grapefruit juice), and vegetables (broccoli, spinach, asparagus, brussels sprouts). Herbal/other plant sources are nettles, alfalfa, parsley, sage, catnip, peppermint, plantain, comfrey leaves, and chickweed.

- *Niacin (B factor)*. Found in grains, meats, and nuts; especially in asparagus, spirulina, cabbage, and bee pollen. Herbal/other plant sources are hops, raspberry leaf, red clover, slippery elm, echinacea, licorice, rose hips, nettles, alfalfa, and parsley.

- *Bioflavonoids*. Found in the pulp and rind of citrus fruits. Herbal/other plant sources are buckwheat greens, blue-green algae, elderberries, hawthorn fruit, rose hips, horsetail, and shepherd's purse.

- *Carotenes*. Found in carrots, cabbage, winter squash, sweet potatoes, green onions, dark leafy greens, apricots, spirulina, and seaweed. Herbal/other plant sources are peppermint, yellow dock, parsley, alfalfa, raspberry leaves, nettles, dandelion greens, kelp, violet leaves, cayenne, paprika, lamb's-quarter, sage, peppermint, chickweed, horsetail, black cohosh, and rose hips.

- *Essential fatty acids (EFAs), including GLA, omega-6, and omega-3*. Found in safflower oil and wheat germ oil. Herbal/other plant sources are all wild plants containing EFAs; flaxseed oil, evening primrose, black currant, and borage.

- *Boron.* Found in organic fruits, vegetables, and nuts. Herbal/other plant sources are all organic weeds, including chickweed, purslane, nettles, dandelion, and yellow dock.

- *Calcium.* Found in milk and dairy products, leafy greens, broccoli, clams, oysters, almonds, walnuts, sunflower seeds, sesame seeds (such as tahini), legumes, tofu, softened bones of canned fish (such as sardines, mackerel, salmon), seaweed, vegetables, whole grains, whey, and shellfish. Herbal/other plant sources are valerian, kelp, nettles, horsetail, peppermint, sage, uva ursi, yellow dock, chickweed, red clover, oat straw, parsley, black currant leaf, raspberry leaf, plantain leaf/seed, borage, dandelion leaf, amaranth leaves, and lamb's-quarter. Depleted by coffee, sugar, salt, alcohol, cortisone enemas, and too much phosphorus in the diet.

- *Chromium.* Found in barley grass, bee pollen, prunes, nuts, mushrooms, liver, beets, and whole-wheat products. Herbal/other plant sources are oat straw, nettles, red clover, catnip, dulse, wild yam, yarrow, horsetail, black cohosh, licorice, echinacea, valerian, and sarsaparilla. Depleted by white sugar.

- *Copper.* Found in liver, shellfish, nuts, legumes, water, organically grown grains, leafy greens, seaweed, and bittersweet chocolate. Herbal/other plant sources are skullcap, sage, horsetail, and chickweed.

- *Iron.* Heme iron (easily absorbed by the body) is found in liver, meat, and poultry; non-heme iron (not as easily absorbed; should be taken with vitamin C) is found in dried fruit, seeds, almonds, cashews, enriched and whole grains, legumes, and green leafy vegetables. Herbal/other plant sources of both types are chickweed, kelp, burdock, catnip, horsetail, Althea root, milk thistle, uva ursi, dandelion leaf/root, yellow dock root, dong quai, black cohosh, echinacea, plantain leaves, sarsaparilla, nettles, peppermint, licorice, valerian, and fenugreek. Depleted by coffee, black tea, enemas, alcohol, aspirin, carbonated drinks, lack of protein, and too much dairy.

- *Magnesium.* Found in leafy greens, seaweed, nuts, whole grains, yogurt, cheese, potatoes, corn, peas, and squash. Herbal/other plant sources are oat straw, licorice, kelp, nettle, dulse, burdock, chickweed, Althea root, horsetail, sage, raspberry leaf, red clover, valerian, yellow dock, dandelion, carrot tops, parsley, and evening primrose. Depleted by alcohol, chemical diuretics, enemas, antibiotics, and excessive fat intake.

- *Manganese.* Found in any leaf or seed from a plant grown in healthy soil and seaweed. Herbal/other plant sources are raspberry leaf, uva ursi, chickweed, milk thistle, yellow dock, ginseng, wild yam, hops, catnip, echinacea, horsetail, kelp, nettles, and dandelion.

- *Molybdenum.* Found in organically raised dairy products, legumes, grains, seaweed, and leafy greens such as kale. Herbal/other plant sources are nettles, dandelion greens, sage, oat straw, fenugreek, raspberry leaves, red clover, horsetail, and chickweed.

- *Nickel.* Found in chocolate, nuts, dried beans, and cereals. Herbal/other plant sources are alfalfa, red clover, oat straw, and fenugreek.

- *Phosphorus.* Found in whole grains, seeds, and nuts. Herbal/other plant sources are peppermint, yellow dock, milk thistle, fennel, hops, chickweed, nettles, dandelion, parsley, dulse, and red clover. Depleted by antacids.

• *Potassium.* Found in celery, cabbage, peas, parsley, broccoli, peppers, carrots, potato skins, eggplant, whole grains, pears, citrus fruits, and seaweeds. Herbal/other plant sources are sage, catnip, hops, dulse, peppermint, skullcap, kelp, red clover, horsetail, nettles, borage, and plantain. Depleted by coffee, sugar, salt, alcohol, enemas, vomiting, diarrhea, chemical diuretics, and dieting.

• *Selenium.* Found in dairy products, seaweed, grains, garlic, liver, kidneys, fish, and shellfish. Herbal/other plant sources are catnip, milk thistle, valerian, dulse, black cohosh, ginseng, uva ursi, hops, echinacea, kelp, raspberry leaf, rose buds and hips, hawthorn fruits, fenugreek, sarsaparilla, and yellow dock.

• *Silicon.* Found in unrefined grains, root vegetables, spinach, and leeks. Herbal/other plant sources are horsetail, dulse, echinacea, cornsilk, burdock, oat straw, licorice, chickweed, uva ursi, and sarsaparilla.

• *Sulfur.* Found in eggs, dairy products, cabbage family plants such as cauliflower and broccoli, onions, garlic, parsley, and watercress. Herbal/other plant sources are nettles, sage, plantain, and horsetail.

• *Zinc.* Found in oysters, seafood, meat, liver, eggs, whole grains, wheat germ, pumpkin seeds, and spirulina. Herbal/other plant sources are skullcap, sage, wild yam, chickweed, echinacea, nettles, dulse, milk thistle, and sarsaparilla. Depleted by alcohol and air pollution.

When to Supplement

Stress depletes the vitamins and minerals in our bodies. Most of us know that the "antistress" vitamins are C (recommended daily intake [RDI] is 4 to 8 grams) and the B vitamins—particularly B_{12} or cobalamin (RDI, 50 to 250 micrograms); B_3 or niacin (RDI, 50 to 150 milligrams); B_6 or pyridoxine (RDI, 50 to 100 milligrams); and B_2 or riboflavin (RDI, 50 to 100 milligrams)—which can be found in a B-complex vitamin supplement. But you should also consider taking these supplements if your diet isn't well balanced; the amounts given are RDIs:

- Beta carotene—10,000 to 25,000 IU
- Bioflavonoids—250 to 500 mg
- Biotin—150 to 500 mcg
- Calcium—600 to 1,000 mg
- Chromium—200 to 400 mcg
- Copper—2 to 3 mg
- Folic acid—500 to 1,000 mcg
- Hydrochloric acid (with meals for chronic stress)—5 to 10 grains
- Inositol—500 to 1,000 mg
- Iodine—150 to 200 mcg
- Iron (menstruating women especially)—10 to 20 mg
- L-amino acids (such as L-glutamine, L-tyrosine, L-phenylalanine, and L-tryptophan)—1,000 to 1,500 mg
- L-cysteine (take with vitamin C)—250 to 500 mg
- Magnesium—350 to 600 mg
- Manganese—5 to 10 mg
- Molybdenum—300 to 800 mg
- Para-aminobenzoic acid (PABA)—50 to 100 mg

- Pancreatic enzymes (after meals) — 1 to 2 tablets
- Pantothenic acid (vitamin B_5) — 500 to 1,000 mg
- Potassium — 300 to 500 mg
- Pyridoxal-5-phosphate — 25 to 75 mg
- Selenium — 200 to 400 mcg
- Sulfur (check with your doctor or pharmacist about RDI)
- Superoxide dismutase (enzyme; check with your doctor or pharmacist about RDI)
- Thiamine (vitamin B_1) 75 to 150 mg
- Vitamin A — 7,500 to 15,000 IU
- Vitamin D — 400 IU
- Vitamin E — 400 to 1,000 IU
- Vitamin K — 200 to 400 mcg
- Water — 2 to 3 quarts
- Zinc — 30 to 60 mg

Carbohydrates and Stress

One of the most important factors in fighting stress is maintaining normal blood sugar levels. Many people suffer from repeated episodes of low blood sugar, known as hypoglycemia. This is usually caused by consuming too many carbohydrates, which produces an initial rush of energy, followed by a tremendous letdown that is sometimes called postprandial (or postmeal) depression. In fact, when we're under stress or feeling depressed, it's not unusual to crave simple carbohydrates such as sugars and sweets. The simpler the carbohydrate, the faster it breaks down into glucose and the faster the subsequent drop in blood sugar, lead-ing to a drop in mood.

If you think you suffer from low blood sugar, schedule an appointment with a nutritionist through your primary care physician and plan a diet that is based on a variety of foods, rather than one that's high in carbohydrates. By increasing your intake of protein and fiber, you can delay the breakdown of food into glucose, which will keep your blood sugar level more stable throughout the day.

Stressful situations can cause us to miss meals or eat on the run, which means we're often eating high-starch foods with very few nutrients. Sitting down at the dining room table or in a restaurant to eat meals, and trying to rest or relax before eating can aid your digestion.

38. Avoid Overeating

Many people overeat when under stress, sometimes to the point of eating compulsively. The following are character-istics of a typical compulsive eater:

- Eating when you're not hungry
- Feeling out of control when you're around food, either trying to resist it or gorging on it
- Spending a lot of time thinking/worrying about food and your weight
- Always being desperate to try another new diet that promises results
- Having feelings of self-loathing and shame
- Hating your body

- Being obsessed with what you can or will eat or have eaten
- Eating in secret or with "eating friends"
- Appearing to others to be a professional dieter who's in control
- Buying cakes or pies as "gifts" and having them wrapped to hide the fact they're for you
- Having a pristine kitchen with only the right foods in it
- Feeling either out of control with food (compulsive eating) or imprisoned by it (dieting)
- Feeling temporary relief by not eating
- Looking forward with pleasure and anticipation to the time when you can eat alone
- Feeling unhappy because of your eating behavior

Most people eat when they're hungry. But if you're a compulsive eater, hunger cues have nothing to do with when you eat. You may eat for any of the following reasons:

- As a social event (This includes family meals and meeting friends at restaurants. You plan food as the social entertainment. Many people do this, but compulsive eaters do it when they're not even hungry.)
- To satisfy mouth hunger—the need to have something in your mouth, even though you're not hungry.
- To prevent future hunger ("Better eat now because I may not get a chance later.")

- As compensation for a bad day or experience or a reward for a good day or experience
- Because you feel it's the only pleasure you can count on
- To calm your nerves
- Because you're bored
- Because you're "going on a diet" tomorrow (Hence, the eating is done out of a real fear that you will be deprived later.)
- Because food is your friend

Food addiction, like other addictions, can be treated successfully with a twelve-step program. The twelve-step theory was started in the 1930s by an alcoholic, who was able to overcome his addiction by essentially saying, "God, help me!" He found other alcoholics who were in a similar position and through an organized, nonjudgmental support system, they overcame their addiction by realizing that God (translated as a higher power, spirit, force, intelligence, or physical properties of the universe) helps those who help themselves. In other words, you have to want help. This is the premise of Alcoholics Anonymous—the most successful existing recovery program for addicts.

People with other addictions have adapted the same basic program using the "Twelve Steps and Twelve Traditions," the founding literature from Alcoholics Anonymous. Overeaters Anonymous (OA) substitutes the phrase "compulsive overeater" for "alcoholic" and "food" for "alcohol." The theme of all twelve-step programs is best expressed through the Serenity Prayer, the first line of which says,

"God, grant me the serenity to accept the things I cannot change, to change the things I can, and the wisdom to know the difference." In other words, you can't take back the food you ate yesterday or last year; but you can control the food you eat today instead of feeling guilty about the past.

39. Practice Yoga

Yoga is not just about stretches or postures; it is actually a way of life. It is part of a whole science of living known as Ayurveda. Ayurveda is an ancient (roughly three thousand years old) Indian approach to health and wellness that has stood up quite well to the test of time. Essentially, it divides up the universe into three basic constitutions, or energies, known as doshas. These doshas are based on wind (vata), fire (pitta), and earth (kapha). They also govern our bodies, personalities, and activities.

When our doshas are balanced, everything functions well, but when they are out of balance, a state of disease (dis-ease as in "not at ease") can set in. Finding the right balance involves changing your diet to suit your predominant dosha (foods are classified as kapha, vata, or pitta, and you eat more or less of whatever you need for balance); practicing yoga, which is a preventive health science that involves certain physical postures and stretches; and meditating. Essentially, yoga is the exercise component of Ayurveda. It involves relaxing meditation, breathing, and physical postures designed to tone and soothe your mental and physical states. Most people find some benefit in taking introductory yoga classes or even following instructional videos.

40. Stretch

Stretching improves muscle blood flow, oxygen flow, and digestion. Therefore, we have a natural desire to stretch. The following stretches will help you relieve tension and achieve a feeling of tranquility:

- While sitting or standing, raise your arms above your head. Keep your shoulders relaxed and breathe deeply for five seconds. Release; repeat five times.

- Gently raise your shoulders in an exaggerated shrug. Breathe deeply and hold for ten seconds. Relax; repeat three times.

- Sit cross-legged on the floor with your spine straight and your neck aligned. Focus on your breath, letting it gently fill the diaphragm and the back of your rib cage. As you inhale, say "So," and as you exhale, say "Hum." Voicing the breath in this manner will keep you focused and relaxed. Continue with "So-Hum" until you feel at ease. (This is the lotus position.)

- Sit on your heels. Bring your forehead to the floor in front of you. Breathe into the back of your rib cage, feeling the stretch in your spine. Hold for as long as it's comfortable.

- Stand tall and find a point across the room on which to focus your gaze. Place the heel of one foot on the opposite inner thigh. Raise your arms above your head until your palms are touching. Breathe deeply, and hold for five seconds. Release; repeat on the other side.

- Lie on your back with palms facing upward, feet turned gently outward. Focus on the movement of breath throughout your body.

- Lie on your belly with arms at your sides. Bend your legs at the knees and bring your heels in toward your buttocks. Reach back and take hold of your right ankle, then your left. Flex your feet if you're having a hard time maintaining this position. Inhale, raising your upper body as far off the floor as possible. Lift your head, completing the arch. Your knees should remain as close together as possible (tying them together might help). Breathe deeply and hold for ten to fifteen seconds.

PART V

Self-Care Strategies

41. Get More Sleep

Sleep deprivation is chronic in our culture, and it is one of the chief aggravators of stress, predisposing you to depression. Lack of sleep increases your levels of cortisol, a stress hormone; depletes your immune system (consuming certain cells you need to destroy viruses and cancerous cells); can promote the growth of fat instead of muscle; and may speed up the aging process.

Normally, cortisol declines before you go to bed as the body's way of preparing for sleep and increases in the morning to wake you up. The hormone is released by the adrenal gland in response to stress and is essentially an "alert" hormone that makes you take action. This is what lets you be sharp-witted in important meetings to close the sale or deal. The cortisol level in your body subsides as the stressful event passes.

A common reason people cut down on their sleep is to get in their workout time before their day begins. For example, it's not unusual for many to rise at 5:00 A.M. in order to get their exercise. This, according to sleep experts, only compromises health and increases stress. The benefits of the health strategies discussed in Part IV may be cancelled out by the harm done through lack of sleep. In the United States, a National Sleep Foundation survey revealed that two out of three people get less than the recommended eight hours of sleep per night; of that group, one out of three get less than six hours of sleep.

There are two phases of sleep: rapid eye movement (REM) and non-rapid eye movement. The first phase, REM, is when researchers believe we dream, an important component in mental health. The non-REM phase is when we experience our deepest sleep, which researchers believe is when various hormones are reset and energy stores are replenished.

Right now, roughly 50 percent of people diagnosed with depression get too much REM sleep and not enough deep sleep. According to a study done at the University of Westminster in London, stress levels are actually lower in people who wake up later than 7:21 A.M.

One way to get more sleep is to schedule nap times into your day. Napping after work for a couple of hours, or during the day if you work from home, can dramatically counter the effects of sleep deprivation. Avoiding alcohol and caffeine before bedtime can also help; instead, try some of the calming herbs discussed in Part IV.

42. Get a Massage

For a lot of people, dramatic emotional wellness is at their fingertips! Massage therapy, technically referred to as soft-tissue manipulation, can be beneficial whether you're receiving the massage from your spouse or a massage therapist trained in any one of dozens of techniques from shiatsu to Swedish massage.

In the East, massage was extensively written about in *The Yellow Emperor's Classic of Internal Medicine*, published in 2700 B.C. (the text that provides the framework for the entire Chinese medicine tradition). Massage is recommended as a treatment for a variety of illnesses.

Swedish massage, the method Westerners are used to, was developed in the nineteenth century by a Swedish doctor and poet, Per Henrik, who borrowed techniques from ancient Egypt, China, and Rome.

The many current forms of massage are based on shiatsu from the East and Swedish massage from the West. Although the philosophies and styles differ in each tradition, the common element is to mobilize the natural healing properties of the body and help it maintain or restore optimal health. Shiatsu-inspired massage focuses on balancing the life force, or life energy. Swedish-inspired massage works on more physiological principles: relaxing muscles to improve blood flow throughout connective tissues, which ultimately strengthens the cardiovascular system.

But no matter what kind of massage you have, there are numerous gliding and kneading techniques used along with deep, circular movements and vibrations that relax your muscles, improve circulation, and increase mobility. This combination is known to help relieve stress and often muscle and joint pain. Added benefits include an improved lymphatic system, faster recovery from musculoskeletal injuries, and reduced edema (water retention).

In fact, a number of employers cover massage therapy in their health plans. Massage is becoming so popular that the number of licensed massage therapists enrolled in the American Message Therapy Association has grown from twelve hundred in 1983 to more than thirty-eight thousand members today. To find a licensed massage therapist, see the Resources section at the back of this book.

Types of massage you may want to investigate include:

- Deep-tissue massage
- Manual lymph drainage
- Neuromuscular massage

- Sports massage
- Swedish massage

43. Meditate

Meditation simply requires you to stop thinking and just be. To do this, people usually find a relaxing spot, sit quietly, and breathe deeply for a few minutes. Going for a nature walk, playing golf, listening to or playing music, reading for pleasure, gardening, listening to silence, or listening only to the sounds of your own breathing are all forms of meditation as well. The point is to give whatever you're doing your full attention and experience it fully.

The following are some other activities that can be meditative:

- Swimming
- Running or jogging
- Walking your dog
- Doing breathing exercises
- Doing stretching exercises
- Practicing yoga or qi gong

44. Find a Place in the Sun

As discussed in Part I, a lack of sunlight can result in seasonal affective disorder (SAD), a form of depression or low mood that is especially common in women. Basically, SAD has many of the features of hibernation—oversleeping and storing up on high fat or carbohydrates for the cold winter—which is good for bears and squirrels, but debilitating for humans.

Women, in particular, need some sunlight to maintain bone health. A little sunlight activates vitamin D in the body, and women have a higher risk for bone loss (osteoporosis) than men. Fifteen minutes of natural sunlight a day is highly recommended for maintaining both bone health and mental health.

But too much sun, without proper protection, can also be hazardous. The following are Sunsense Guidelines from the American and Canadian Cancer Societies:

• Reduce sun exposure between 11 A.M. and 4 P.M., when the sun's rays are the strongest. If you can, plan your outdoor activities before or after this time. An easy way to remember this rule is that during these hours, your shadow is shorter than you are!

• Seek shade or create your own. When you are outside, especially during the middle of the day, try to stay in the shade. Be prepared for places without any shade by taking along an umbrella. That way you can create shade wherever you need it.

• Slip on clothing to cover your arms and legs. Covering your skin will protect it from the sun. Choose clothes that are loose fitting, tightly woven, and lightweight.

• Slap on a wide-brimmed hat. Most skin cancers occur on the face and neck, so these areas need extra protection. Wear a hat with a wide brim that covers your entire head and neck. Hats without a wide brim, like baseball caps, don't give you enough protection.

• Slop on a sunscreen with sun protection factor (SPF) 15 or higher. Look for the words *broad spectrum* on the label. This means the product offers protection against two types of ultraviolet rays, UV-A and UV-B. Apply sunscreen generously twenty minutes before outdoor activities. Reapply frequently—at least every two hours—and after swimming or exercise that makes you perspire. Remember that no sunscreen can absorb all of the sun's rays. Use it along with shade, clothing, and hats—not instead of them.

• Babies need extra sun protection because their skin is very sensitive. Keep infants under one year out of direct sunlight, and place your child's stroller or playpen in the shade.

• Don't think that tanning parlors and sunlamps are substitutes for the sun. They do not give you a "safe tan without burning." No tan is a safe tan; it's evidence of skin damage. Just like the sun, tanning lights and sunlamps emit ultraviolet rays that can cause sunburn, age skin, and increase your risk of skin cancer. The strength of the ultraviolet rays, especially the UV-A type, may actually be higher in a tanning bed than in sunlight!

• Wear sunglasses. They can help prevent damage to your eyes by blocking a large amount of ultraviolet rays. Keep your shades on, and make sure your children wear them, too. Choose sunglasses with even shading, medium to dark lenses (gray, brown, or green tint), and UV-A and UV-B protection. These qualities can be found even in many inexpensive sunglasses.

• Check your skin regularly. Most skin cancers can be cured if caught early enough. Get to know your skin. Know the location and appearance of birthmarks and moles, and examine them regularly so you can detect any changes. See your doctor right away if you notice any of the following:

A birthmark or mole that changes shape, color, size, or texture

A sore that does not heal

New growths on your skin

Patches of skin that bleed, ooze, swell, itch, or become red or bumpy

45. Consider Counseling

From time to time, one of the best things you can do to solve a problem is consult a professional. Simply talking to an objective listener can make an enormous difference.

Types of Professionals

Most people looking for sorting-out-your-life counseling do well with counselors or social workers, but the following professionals can all help.

Psychologist and Psychological Associate

This is someone who can be licensed to practice therapy with either a master's degree or doctoral degree. Clinical psychologists have a Master of Science (M.S.) or Master of Arts (M.A.) degree and usually work in a hospital or clinic setting, although they often can be found in private practice as well. They may also hold a Doctor of Philosophy (Ph.D.) in psychology, a Doctor of Education (Ed.D.), or a Doctor of Psychology (Psy.D.).

Social Worker

This professional holds a Bachelor of Social Work (B.S.W.) and/or a Master of Social Work (M.S.W.) degree with a bachelor's degree in another discipline (which is not uncommon). Some social workers have doctoral degrees as well. All social workers must meet individual state legal requirements to be designated a certified social worker (CSW). The National Association of Social Workers (NASW) has its own, nongovernmental credentialing program, which confers membership in the Academy of Certified Social Workers (ACSW). Unlike the CSW, which (in most states) requires graduation from a master's level program and a state board exam, the ACSW requires two years of supervised experience following graduation from a master's program. Social workers who include a *P* and *R* in their credentials are qualified under state law to receive insurance reimbursement for outpatient services to clients with group health insurance. *P* indicates the CSW has had three years of supervised experience, while *R* indicates six years. Each initial refers to different types of insurance policies.

Psychiatric Nurse

This is most likely a registered nurse (R.N.) with a Bachelor of Science in Nursing (B.S.N.) and a master's degree (either an M.A. or an M.S.), although neither degree is required. This type of nurse has done most of her training in a psychiatric setting and may be trained in the field of psychotherapy.

Counselor

This professional has usually completed certification courses in counseling and obtained a license to practice psychotherapy; he or she may have, but does not require, a college degree. Frequently, though, counselors have a master's degree in a related field, such as social work. Or their degree may be in a field that has nothing to do with mental health. The term *professional counselor* is used for people who have earned the minimum of a master's degree and possess professional knowledge and demonstrable skills in the application of mental health, psychological, and human development principles in order to facilitate human development and adjustment throughout the life span.

As of January 1999, the District of Columbia and forty-four states had enacted some type of counselor credentialing law to regulate the use of titles related to the counseling profession. The abbreviations CPC (certified professional counselor) and LPC (licensed professional counselor) indicate credentials granted by the state. No matter what letters you see, however, it's always a good idea to ask your counselor what training he or she has had in the field of mental health.

Marriage and Family Counselor

This is somewhat different than the broader term *counselor*. This professional has completed rigorous training through certification courses in family therapy and relationship dynamics, and has obtained a license to practice psychotherapy. He or she should have the designations MFT (Master of Family Therapy) or AAMFT (American Association for Marriage and Family Therapy). A MFT has graduate training (a master's or doctoral degree) in marriage and family therapy and at least two years of clinical experience. Forty-one states currently license, certify, or regulate MFTs.

Styles of Therapy

There are a range of therapy techniques used in stress counseling. Here are some of the more common ones.

Cognitive-Behavioral Therapy

This method is oriented toward having an upbeat attitude and correcting what is referred to as disordered thinking (dwelling on negative thoughts). The premise is that how you think can affect how you feel. For example, if a friend cancels a lunch date with you, or somebody doesn't return your phone call or E-mail, you may take it personally and make assumptions that he or she doesn't like you. That thought then leads you to feel badly about yourself, reinforcing feelings of low self-esteem or even self-loathing and creating a downward spiral.

A cognitive-behavioral therapist will ask you to consider other reasons for the cancellation or unreturned call. Perhaps the other person has overwhelming problems that have absolutely nothing to do with you. Perhaps a last-minute deadline came up, or problems and stresses in his or her personal life necessitated the cancellation. In other words, not everything you perceive to be negative is really negative, and not everything you take personally is really personal.

Ultimately, if you think negative thoughts about yourself and believe you're a failure or that your life is doomed, you are more apt to be sad. On the other hand, if you think positive thoughts and believe in yourself, you are more apt to be happy. Although this might sound like an easy, quick-fix approach, changing your perspective on life can be powerful. However, in the midst of depression, this technique may have limited success. Essentially, what's past is past, and you can decide *today* to be a more positive person, which in turn, can attract more positive experiences into your life.

Interpersonal Therapy

This is a very specific approach based on the idea that malfunctioning relationships contribute to the emotional symptoms of stress. You and your therapist will explore your current relationships and recent events that may have affected those relationships, such as loss, conflict, or possible lifestyle changes. You may also explore the roles various people play in your life, what your expectations of them are, and vice versa. Your therapist works in a supportive role to help you develop better strategies to cope or negotiate with key people in your life, which in turn helps to resolve conflicts. Much of this has to do with setting reasonable expectations for relationships and looking at how you may have misinterpreted the actions of others to reflect badly on them or yourself.

Psychodynamic Therapy

This technique deals with the ghosts of relationships and events from your past, the dynamics of your upbringing, and present events and relationships. Here, your thoughts, emotions, and behavior over a lifetime are examined; patterns of behavior and aspects of your personality are discussed as possible sources of both internal and external conflict. Couples or group therapy is often involved in this type of therapy. The adage "the past is history, the future a mystery, and the present a gift" works well in this context.

Finding a Therapist

There are some hallmarks of good therapists that you should be aware of as you're looking for one you like:

• *Exhibiting genuine caring.* Your therapist should demonstrate a basic concern for your welfare, the ability to empathize, and the ability to communicate that empathy.

• *Accepting your criticism.* If you get angry or critical, your therapist shouldn't take it personally and should be able to accept valid criticism well. You need to feel sure that you can sound off in a session without your therapist holding it against you or retaliating somehow. (A therapist should feel free to interpret your anger, if your criticism is not valid.)

• *Giving you reliable service and undivided attention.* Your therapist should not frequently cancel sessions; change session times; take phone calls during sessions; or use your time to discuss fees, payments, and so on. Nor should your therapist cut you off in the middle of an epiphany because your time's up. (Epiphanies don't happen every day; they should be respected.) That said, you shouldn't take advantage of your therapist and try to manipulate him or her for more time. Obviously, if a therapist cannot give you an extra minute now and then, there's a problem. But there are clients who overstep the boundary and continuously run overtime, which interferes with someone else's time. And that's not fair, either.

• *Refraining from discussing his or her own problems.* Your therapist isn't your hairdresser; it's not tit-for-tat. You shouldn't be expected to listen to his or her personal problems during your sessions.

• *Practicing within a code of ethics.* Your therapist should keep your sessions confidential; your sessions should not be tape recorded, videotaped, or staged in front of a one-way mirror behind which his or her colleagues are watching without your knowledge. Any time your session is recorded or observed by others (which may be the case if the therapist is in training, is training someone else, or would like to consult with someone else about your case), it must be done with your full consent. Otherwise, you cannot trust your therapist and should find help elsewhere.

46. Pamper Yourself

Taking care of yourself means being good to yourself. Give yourself some tender loving care. You'll find this goes a long way toward battling daily stresses. Here are some suggestions:

• Set aside "comfort time" for yourself at least once a week. Make it a ritual. Having coffee with your morning paper; taking a scenic stroll or window-shopping in a favorite neighborhood; taking a long bath; going to an open market (often held on the weekends), or having breakfast in bed once a week are all feel-good activities that will make you feel energized and loved.

• Have a very long shower each morning. Treat yourself to a shower massage and take the time to massage every part of your body. Buy energizing shower gels or shower toys to use each day.

• Have a steam bath. Run the shower, sit in your bathroom on a mat, and just enjoy the steam.

• Have a luxurious bubble bath. Using aromatherapy to augment your bath can work wonders to relieve stress. For a spa-style bath, use a mud product, dried milk powder for a milk bath, or mineral salts for aching muscles. The bath ritual can be enhanced with candlelight and body oils or lotions to moisturize afterward.

• Take a bed-rest day. Change the linens; fluff up your pillows; stock up on good reading material; get a tray of favorite snacks, wine, coffee or tea, and so on; and go to bed. Count it as a sick day and rejuvenate.

• Plan a spa day (again, take it as a sick day if you like). Start your day with a bubble bath, as described earlier. Then go outside for a nice, long walk. When you get back, take an invigorating shower, scrubbing your body with a loofah or rough washcloth. Wash your hair and put in a conditioning treatment. After your shower, give yourself a pedicure while you run another bath with essential oils (see section 36 in the previous chapter). Cleanse your face well and apply your favorite facial mask. Light some candles and soak; put a cool washcloth or cucumber slices over your eyes. When you're done, get back in the shower and rinse off the mask. Remoisturize your body. Wrap yourself in a towel and take a nap. (You may want to arrange in advance for a massage therapist to visit you at this point!) After your nap, make a smoothie with your favorite fruits. To top off the day, order in from your favorite restaurant. Go to bed early with a book or magazine and a tray of snacks or leftovers.

47. Cry More, Laugh More, and Learn to Forgive

Releasing emotions uses up stress hormones and gets them out of your system. One of the best ways to do this is by having a good cry. Human tears contain high levels of stress hormone, which is one reason people who cry tend to have less stress than those who do not. If you need something to get you sobbing, try a dramatic movie (there's a reason we call them tear-jerkers) to help induce tears. Laughter is another way of relieving stress because it makes you feel good, which boosts your levels of endorphins—the proteins that combat stress hormones. Laughter also creates deep muscle relaxation (which is why you can sometimes lose bladder control). Your blood pressure also drops, while the T cells in your immune system increase. Incorporating humor into your life can be fun, too. Look for humorous books, magazines, or other materials and keep them handy. Subscribe to a humor listserv (but not if it creates E-stress; see Part III). Rent funny videos; watch comedy shows and networks, and use laughter to defuse stress in the office or at home. Laughter bonds people together and attracts others to you. Teachers, doctors, and salespeople who generate laughter have more loyal students, more compliant patients, and higher sales!

The final great defense against depression is forgiveness. When you have unresolved conflict with someone or you're nursing a grudge, the emotional weight you carry when you think about the situation increases blood pressure, stress hormones, heart rate, perspiration, and muscle tension. Forgiveness doesn't mean excusing bad behavior, but it does mean you are prepared to move forward and let go of your bitterness toward the other person. Forgiveness is healthier for you, and chances are the person with whom you are in conflict would either welcome your forgiveness or, deep down, wants to forgive you as well.

Forgiveness is about saying the Serenity Prayer (accepting the things you cannot change, changing the things you can). You can't change the fact that the conflict occurred, but you can change your current response to it. Among the things you cannot change are:

- Other people
- Your age
- The way you were raised
- A death, illness, or accident in the family
- Being laid off from a job

You can change the following:

- Your reaction to others
- Your goals
- Your self-esteem and self-worth
- How you treat others
- How you treat yourself
- Your willingness to communicate your needs to others

48. Look into Pressure Point Therapies

Pressure point therapies involve using the fingertips to apply pressure to specific points on the body that are believed to help reduce stress, anxiety, pain, and other physical symptoms of stress and other ailments. There are different kinds of pressure point therapies; the most well known are acupuncture and reflexology.

Acupuncture is an ancient Chinese healing art that aims to restore the smooth flow of life energy (*qi*) in your body. Acupuncturists believe that your *qi* can be accessed from various points on your body, such as your ear. Each point is also associated with a specific organ. Depending on what's bothering you, an acupuncturist will insert a very fine needle at a specific point to restore *qi* to various organs. Each of the roughly two thousand points on your body has a specific therapeutic effect when stimulated, and it's now believed that acupuncture stimulates the release of endorphins, which is why it's effective at reducing stress, pain, and so forth. *Jin shin jyutsu* and *jin shin do* are other pressure point therapies similar to acupuncture.

Although reflexology originated in the East, Western reflexology was developed by Dr. William Fitzgerald—an American ear, nose, and throat specialist—who talked about this technique as "zone therapy." In fact, reflexology is popular in several cultures, including those in Egypt, India, Africa, China, and Japan. In the same way that Chinese medicine uses the ears as a map to the organs, the feet play the same role in reflexology. By applying pressure to certain parts of the hands, ears, and most widely known— feet—reflexologists can ease pain and tension and restore the body's life force.

Like most Eastern healing arts, reflexology focuses on releasing the flow of energy through the body along its various pathways. When this energy is trapped for some reason, illness can result. When the energy is released, the body can begin to heal itself. A reflexologist views the foot as a microcosm of the entire body. Individual reference points or reflex areas correspond to all major organs, glands, and parts of the body. Applying pressure to a specific area of the foot stimulates the movement of energy to the corresponding body part.

Shiatsu massage also involves using pressure points. A healer using shiatsu will move along the length of each energy pathway (also called meridians), applying thumb pressure to successive points along the way. The aim is to stimulate acupressure points while giving you some of the healer's life energy. Barefoot shiatsu involves the healer using his or her foot instead of the hand to apply pressure. You can learn to massage your own pressure points. Here are some simple exercises you can try:

• With the thumb of one hand, slowly work your way across the palm of the other hand, from the base of the little finger to the base of the index finger. Then rub the center of your palm with your thumb. Push on this point; this will calm your nervous system. Repeat this on the other hand.

• To relieve a headache, grasp the flesh at the base of one thumb with the opposite index finger and thumb. Squeeze gently and massage the tissue in a circular motion. Then pinch each fingertip. Switch to the other hand.

• For general stress relief, find sore pressure points on your feet and ankles. Gently press your thumb into them, and massage each point. The tender areas indicate stress in particular parts of your body. By rubbing them, you're relieving the tension in the corresponding organs, glands, and tissues. You can also apply pressure with bunched or extended fingers, your knuckles, the heel of your hand, or a gripping motion.

• Use the same effective technique for self-massage on your hands, looking for tender points on the palms and wrists.

• Massage your ears. Feel for tender spots and rub them vigorously. Within about four minutes, your ears will get very hot.

49. Ask for Support from Family or Friends

When you're feeling under great stress or are simply going through a bad time, ask family or friends for some help. Knowing that things won't fall apart can be the source of greatest comfort when you feel overwhelmed. Unfortunately, too many people are treated to family harassment in the sense that they are not given the space to go through bad days. Constantly being told "Snap out of it," "Get out of the house," or "What you need is a nice cup of tea (or soup, hot chocolate, etc.)" isn't support. But when family or friends look after as many of the meals, chores, and so on as they can, it takes pressure off of you. You may have trouble asking for help and then worry about how to get everything done, which only adds to your burden.

Allow yourself some time with close family or friends to unburden yourself. Taking some time to discuss things that are bothering you is a form of self-care. Your loved ones will be able to offer unique support and advice in certain situations because they are familiar with the players in your drama. Always hiding your troubles or trying to act as though everything is perfect just places more stress on you.

50. Eliminate Anxiety Triggers

Anxiety can trigger or accompany bouts of depression. Do yourself a favor and cut down (or cut out) some of the following.

Caffeine

I'll make this short and sweet. Lots of studies show that caffeine causes anxiety and sleeplessness and is mildly addictive. Experts now recommend that you consume no more than 400 to 500 milligrams of caffeine per day, which is equal to two 8-ounce mugs of regular coffee or four cups of instant coffee. Of course, there are many other sources of caffeine, such as soft drinks, chocolate, tea, and so forth. All of them should be taken into account when calculating your daily intake.

Smoking

Many people turn to cigarettes to deal with the demands of stress, but those who smoke every day are twice as likely to suffer from depression as people who don't smoke. This may have nothing to do with smoking and everything to do with stressful circumstances. In other words, people under a lot of stress are more likely to suffer from depression, and a lot of those people are likely to smoke to try to calm themselves. Studies have found that people with major depression are three times as likely to be daily smokers, and nicotine may be a drug we crave to medicate our depressed moods.

Alcohol

If you tend to have wine or other alcoholic beverages to unwind after a stressful day, be aware that alcohol can interfere with sleep patterns and also is a depressant. Initially, it may make you feel tired, so you believe it's a sleeping aid; but it can wake you up later on, leaving you wide awake at 2:00 A.M. and preventing you from going back to sleep. Naturally, all of this can aggravate stress and fatigue.

Some interesting things for women to note: Women metabolize alcohol differently than men, so even when a man and woman are the same weight, the woman will become intoxicated more easily than the man. This has to do with the way body fat is distributed. The same woman will also tolerate alcohol differently at different times in her menstrual cycle. She may become more easily intoxicated just before ovulation, which can aggravate symptoms of PMS. Women also tend to be invisible drinkers (drinking alone).

Moderate drinking is defined as fewer than twelve drinks per week and is not a daily activity. Moderate drinkers do not use alcohol to cope with stress, nor do they plan their recreational activities around alcohol. If you think you're drinking more heavily than you used to, keeping a diary of how much you drink and when is useful. Often, just being aware of your alcohol consumption patterns can be enough to change your habits.

Diet

When you're stressed and fatigued, you often don't eat well. By eating properly—meaning a variety of foods, particularly all vegetables—you'll be in better shape to cope. (See Part IV.)

Conclusion

Over the years, I've written extensively about depression and spoken to many people who have suffered from it. They have asked me to provide information about preventing depression without the use of strong medication, which often has debilitating side effects. This book is my response to that request. You now have in your hands fifty ways to not only prevent and fight depression without having to use drugs, but also to reduce your risk of virtually every illness, since the precursors to depression—stress and anxiety—can predispose us to autoimmune diseases, cancers, heart disease, stroke, and viral and bacterial infections. By incorporating just one idea from this book into your life you may be able to prevent recurring bouts of depression, if you've struggled with it in the past, or even prevent depression from entering your life altogether.

Resources

Counseling

The Alliance for the Mentally Ill/Friends and Advocates of the Mentally Ill (AMI/FAMI)
    432 Park Avenue South #710
    New York, NY 10016-8013
    Help line: (212) 684-FAMI; office: (212) 684-3365;
    Events line: (212) 684-4237

American Association of Marriage and Family Therapy
    1133 15th Street, NW, Suite 300
    Washington, DC 20005-2710
    Phone: (202) 452-0109
    Website: aamft.org

American Counseling Association
    5999 Stevenson Avenue
    Alexandria, VA 22304
    Phone: (703) 823-9800
    Website: counseling.org

American Psychological Association
  Office of Public Affairs
  750 First Street, NE
  Washington, DC 20002-4242
  Phone: (202) 336-5700
  Website: apa.org

Center for Cognitive Therapy
  3600 Market Street, 8th Floor
  Philadelphia, Pennsylvania 19104-2649
  Phone: (215) 898-4100

Depression Awareness, Recognition and Treatment
(D/ART) Program
  National Institute of Mental Health
  Phone: (800) 421-4211 or (301) 443-4140

Depressives Anonymous: Recovery from Depression
  329 E. 62nd Street
  New York, NY 10021
  Phone: (212) 689-2600

Foundation for Depression and Manic Depression
  24 E. 81st Street
  New York, NY 10028
  Phone: (212) 772-3400

Freedom from Fear
  308 Seaview Avenue
  Staten Island, NY 10305
  Phone: (718) 351-1717; fax: (718) 667-8893

Freedom from Fear is a not-for-profit organization acting as advocate for those suffering from anxiety and depressive disorders.

Jonathan O. Cole Mental Health Consumer
Resource Center
    McLean Hospital,
    115 Mill Street, Rehab. 113
    Belmont, MA 02178
    Phone: (617) 855-3298 or 2795; fax: (617) 855-3666

Justice in Mental Health Organization United States
of America
    421 Seymour Street
    Lansing, MI 48933
    Phone: (517) 371-2266

National Alliance for the Mentally Ill (NAMI)
    200 North Glebe Road #1015
    Arlington, VA 22201-3754
    Help line: (800) 950-NAMI; office: (703) 524-7600;
    fax: (703) 524-9094
    Website: nami.org

The National Association of Social Workers (NASW)
    750 First Street, NE, Suite 700
    Washington, DC 20002-4241
    Phone: (202) 408-8600; fax: (202) 336-8311; TDD:
    (202) 408-8396
    Website (for a list of chapter offices): naswdc.org.

National Depressive and Manic-Depressive Association
    730 North Franklin Street, Suite 501
    Chicago, IL 60610
    Phone: (800) 82-NDMDA or (312) 642-0049; fax:
    (312) 642-7243

National Institute of Mental Health (NIMH)
   Public Inquiries
   6001 Executive Boulevard, Rm. 8184, MSC 9663
   Bethesda, MD 20892-9663
   Phone: (301) 443-4513; fax: (301) 443-4279
   E-mail: nimhinfo@nih.gov; website: nimh.nig.gov

National Institute of Mental Health, Panic
Disorder Division
   Panic Disorder Education Program
   Room 7C-02, Fishers Lane
   Rockville, MD 20857
   Phone: (800) 64-PANIC

National Mental Health Association
   1021 Prince Street
   Alexandria, VA 22314-2971
   Phone: (800) 969-6642 or (703) 684-7722
   Website: healthtouch.com

World Federation for Mental Health
   1021 Prince Street
   Alexandria, VA 22314-2971
   Phone: (703) 684-7722

Body Work/Hands-On Healing

American Academy of Medical Acupuncture
   5820 Wilshire Boulevard, Suite 500
   Los Angeles, CA 90036
   Phone: (800) 521-2262
   Website: medicalacupuncture.org

American Academy of Osteopathy
   3500 DePauw Boulevard, Suite 1080
   Indianapolis, IN 46268-1136
   Phone: (317) 879-1881

American Academy of Reflexology
606 E. Magnolia Boulevard, Suite B
Burbank, CA 91501-2618
Phone: (818) 841-7741

American Chiropractic Association
1701 Clarendon Boulevard
Arlington, VA 22209
Phone: (703) 276-8800

American Massage Therapy Association
820 Davis Street, Suite 100
Evanston, IL 60201-4444
Phone: (847) 864-0123; fax: (847)864-1178
E-mail: infor@inet.amtamassage.org; website:
amtamassage.org

American Osteopathic Association
142 E. Ontario Street
Chicago, IL 60611
Phone: (800) 621-1773 or (312) 280-5800
Website: am-osteo-assn.org

Association for Network Chiropractic
444 N. Main Street
Longmont, CO 80501
Phone: (303) 678-8086

International Chiropractors Association
1110 N. Glebe Road, Suite 1000
Arlington, VA 22201
Phone: (703) 528-5000
E-mail: chiro@erols.com; website: chiropractic.org

International Institute of Reflexology
    Box 12462
    St. Petersburg, FL 33733
    Phone: (813) 343-4811
    E-mail: ftreflex@concentric.net

Jin Shin Do Foundation for Bodymind Acupressure
    1048G San Miguel Canyon Road
    Watsonville, CA 95076
    Phone: (408) 763-1551

Jin Shin Jyutsu, Inc.
    8719 E. San Alberto Drive
    Scottsdale, AZ 85258
    Phone: (602) 998-9331; fax: (602) 998-9335

National Center for Complementary and
Alternative Medicine
    National Institutes of Health
    8630 Fenton Street, Suite 1130
    Silver Spring, MD 20910
    Phone: (888) 644-6226
    Website: nccam.nih.gov

National Certification Board of Therapeutic
Massage and Bodywork
    8201 Greensboro Drive, Suite 300
    McLean, VA 22102
    Phone: (800) 296-0664 or (703) 610-9015; fax: (703)
    610-9005
    Website: ncbtmb.com

North American Society of Teachers of the
Alexander Technique
    3010 Hennepin Avenue S, Suite 10
    Minneapolis, MN 55408
    Phone: (800) 473-0620 or (612) 824-5066

Nurse Healers — Professional Associates, Inc.
175 Fifth Avenue, Suite 2755
New York, NY 10010
Phone: (212) 886-3776

Office of Alternative Medicine Clearinghouse
Box 8218
Silver Spring, MD 20907-8218
Phone: (888) 644-6226
Website: http://altmed.od.nih.gov
For information about federally sponsored research in manual therapies

Rolf Institute of Structural Integration
205 Canyon Boulevard
Boulder, CO 80302
Phone: (800) 530-8875
E-mail: rolfinst@aol.com; website: rolf.org

The Feldenkrais Guild
524 Ellsworth Street, Box 489
Albany, OR 97321-0143
Phone: (800) 775-2118 or (541) 926-0572
E-mail:feldngld@peak.org; website: feldenkrais.com

The New Center College for Wholistic Health Education
& Research
6801 Jericho Turnpike
Syosset, NY 11791
Phone: (800) 922-7337 or (516) 364-5533; fax: (516) 364-0989
E-mail: newcenter@d.com; website: newcenter.edu

TRAGER Institute
   21 Locust Avenue
   Mill Valley, CA 94941
   Phone: (415) 388-2688
   E-mail: admin@trager.com; website: trager.com

Chronic Fatigue Syndrome

The CFIDS Association of America, Inc.
   P.O. Box 220398
   Charlotte, NC 28222-0398
   Phone: (800) 442-3437 (44-CFIDS) or (704)
   362-2343; fax: (704) 365-9755
   E-mail: info@cfids.org

Allergy Asthma Information Center & Hotline
   P.O. Box 1766
   Rochester, NY 14603
   Phone: (800) 727-5400

American Academy of Allergy and Immunology
   611 E. Wells Street
   Milwaukee, WI 53202
   Phone: (800) 822-2762

American Chronic Pain Association
   P.O. Box 850
   Rocklin, CA 95677
   Phone: (916) 632-0922

American College of Allergy and Immunology
   800 E. Northwest Highway, Suite 1080
   Palatine, IL 60067-6516
   Phone: (800) 842-7777

CFIDS Activation Network (CAN)
P.O. Box 345
Larchmont, NY 10538
Phone: (212) 627-5631

CFS Crisis Center
27 W. 20th Street, Suite 703
New York, NY 10011
Phone: (212) 691-4800; fax: (212) 691-5113

Chemical Injury Information Network
P.O. Box 301
White Sulphur Springs, MT 59645-0301
Phone: (406) 547-2255

Chicago CFS Association
818 Wenonah Avenue
Oak Park, IL 60304
Phone: (708) 524-9322

The Connecticut CFIDS Association
P.O. Box 9582
Forestville, CT 06011
Phone: (203) 582-3437 (582-CFIDS)

Sensitive to a Toxic Environment (STATE)
The STATE Foundation
P.O. Box 834
Orchard Park, NY 14127
Phone: (716) 675-1164

For people with multiple chemical sensitivities

National CFIDS Foundation
103 Aletha Road
Needham, MA 02492
Phone: (781) 449-3535; fax: (781) 449-8606 or (781) 925-3393

National CFS & Fibromyalgia Association
P.O. Box 18426
Kansas City, MO 64133
Phone: (816) 313-2000

Fibromyalgia Network
5700 Stockdale Highway, Suite 100
Bakersfield, CA 93309
Phone: (805) 631-1950 (from 10 A.M. to 2 P.M.
Pacific time)

American Academy of Environmental Medicine
P.O. Box 16106
Denver, CO 80216
Phone: (303) 622-9755

Additional Links

- American Association of Marriage and Family Therapy: amft.org

- American Association of Suicidology: suicidology.org

- American Counseling Association: counseling.org

- American Psychiatric Association: psych.org

- American Psychological Association: apa.org

- Anxiety Disorders Association of America: adaa.org

- Association of Gay and Lesbian Psychologists (AGLP): psy.uva.nl

- AtHealth.com (mental health links, chat, bulletin board, etc.): athealth.com

- Canadian Mental Health Association: cmha.ca

- CFS Days (for sufferers of chronic fatigue syndrome and fibromyalgia; information about signs and symptoms, research, diagnosis, treatment and medications; discussion and support group): sunflower.org/~cfsdays/cfsdays.htm

- Chronic Fatigue Syndrome at About.com: http://chronicfatigue/.about.com/health/chronicfatigu e/mbody.htm

- Depression Knowledge Center (put together by the World Federation for Mental Health, a very comprehensive site that offers FAQs, events listings, lists of organizations, archives, and discussion): depressionnet.org

- International Society for Mental Health: ismh.org

- Internet Mental Health (information on disorders and treatment, with online diagnostic services and psychopharmacology index): mentalhealth.com

- Mental health at About.com (updated daily with articles, forums, chat, and a newsletter): mentalhealth.about.com

- Mental Health Center (answers to many of the questions you're too scared to ask): mentalhealthcenter.com

- Mental Health Links (web directory of useful links, associations, news and events, support, self-help, and managed care): mentalhealthlinks.com

- Mental Help (award-winning guide to mental health, psychology, and psychiatry): mentalhelp.net

- National Alliance for the Mentally Ill (NAMI): nami.org

- National Association of Social Workers (NASW): naswdc.org
- National Center for Post Traumatic Stress Disorder (PTSD): dartmouth.edu/dms/ptsd
- National Institute of Mental Health (NIMH): nimh.nig.gov
- National Mental Health Association: healthtouch.com
- Obsessive Compulsive Foundation: http://pages.prodigy.com/alwillen.ocf.html
- Online Dictionary of Mental Health: shef.as.ulc/~psyc/psychotherapy/index
- Society for Light Treatment and Biological Rhythms (for SAD sufferers): websciences.org/sltbr
- Walkers (information, a forum, and chat rooms for depressives and their loved ones): walkers.org

For more information about disease prevention and wellness, visit me online at sarahealth.com, where you will find over three hundred links for good health and wellness.

Bibliography

Allardice, Pamela. *Essential Oils: The Fragrant Art of Aromatherapy.* Vancouver: Raincoast Books, 1999.

American Institute of Stress. "America's #1 health problem." *The International Journal of Stress Management.* Retrieved from stress.org, June 15, 2001.

Antibiotics in Animals: An Interview with Stephen Sundlof, D.V.M., Ph.D., 1997. International Food Information Council, 1100 Connecticut Avenue N.W., Suite 430, Washington, D.C. 20036.

"Antidepressants' impact mainly from boost of getting treated, study suggests." The Associated Press, electronic news service, July 20, 1998.

Baker, Sandy. "The number one way to eliminate daily stress." *The National Public Account* Dec 1000; 44(10):13.

Ballweg, Rachel. "Seven simple ways to reduce stress." *Better Homes and Gardens,* Jan 2000; 78(1):62.

Ben-Ari, Elia T. "Take two exercise sessions and call me in the morning." *BioScience,* Jan 2000; 50(1):96.

———. "Walking the tightrope between work and family." *BioScience,* May 2000; 50(5):472.

Bennetts, Leslie. "e-Stress." *FamilyPC*, June 2000; 7(6):93.

Bowen, Jon. "Fisticuffs in the cube: Stressed-out office workers are succumbing to 'desk rage.'" Retrieved from salon.com., September 7, 1999.

Bower, Peter J., et al. "Manual therapy: Hands-on healing." *Patient Care*, 15 Dec 1997; 31(20):69.

Canadian Cancer Society. *Sunsense Guidelines*, 2000. Canadian Cancer Society, Toronto.

Carlson, Betty Clark. "Managing time for personal effectiveness: Achieving goals with less stress." *ISMA-USA Newsletter* Spring 1999; 1(1):1-2.

Carlson, John G. "Relax Your Way to Stress Management." International Stress Management Association. Retrieved from stress.org, June 2000.

Cass, Hyla. *St. John's Wort: Nature's Blues Buster*. New York: Avery Publishing Group, 1998.

Chaddock, Brenda. "Activity is key to diabetes health." *Canadian Pharmacy Journal* Mar 1997:14.

———. "Foul weather fitness: The hardest part is getting started." *Canadian Pharmacy Journal* Mar 1996:42.

———. "The Magic of Exercise." *Canadian Pharmacy Journal* Sept 1995:45.

Christmas Derrick, Rachel. "Less stress on the job." *Essence*, Mar 2000; 30(11):44.

Cicala, Roger S. *The Heart Disease Sourcebook*. Lowell House, 1998. Los Angeles.

Clarke, Bill. "Action figures." *Diabetes Dialogue*, Fall 1996; 43(3):14–16.

Clarke, Robyn D. "Serenity now." *Black Enterprise*, Jan 2000; 30(6):115.

"Combat job stress: Does work make you sick?" Retrieved from: convoke.com/markjr/cjstress.html, February 12, 1999.

Controlling Anger Before It Controls You. National Mental Health Association, 1996.

Costin, Carolyn. *The Eating Disorder Sourcebook.* Los Angeles: Lowell House, 1996.

Cotton, Paul. "Environmental estrogenic agents area of concern." *JAMA* 9 Feb 1994; 271:414, 416.

Curtis, Patricia. "Stress-free zone." *Redbook*, June 2000:194(6):157.

Dadd, Debra Lynn. *The Nontoxic Home and Office.* Los Angeles: Jeremy P. Tarcher, 1992.

Datao, Robert. *The Law of Stress.* The International Stress Management Association, June 2000.

Davis, Martha, Elizabeth Robbins Eshelman, and Matthew McKay. *The Relaxation and Stress Reduction Workbook.* Oakland, CA: New Harbinger, 1995.

Delanet, Kathy, and Marie R. Squillace. *Living with Heart Disease*, Los Angeles: Lowell House, 1998.

Douglas, Ann. *Sanity Savers: The Canadian Working Woman's Guide to (Almost) Having It All.* Toronto: McGraw-Hill Ryerson, 1999.

Dreher, Henry, and Alice D. Domar. *Healing Mind, Healthy Woman.* New York: Henry Holt and Co., 1996.

Eighth Biennial Report on Great Lakes Water Quality, Under the Great Lakes Water Quality Agreement of 1978 to the Governments of the United States and Canada and the State and Provincial Governments of the Great Lakes Basin, 1996. International Joint Commission, 1250 23rd Street NW, Suite 100, Washington, D.C., 20440.

Engel, June V. "Beyond vitamins: Phytochemicals to help fight disease." *Health News*, June 1996:14.

Evans, Julie A. "Stop back pain instantly!" *Prevention*, July 1999; 51(7):128.

Everyday Carcinogens: Stopping Cancer Before It Starts. Proceedings from the Workshop on Primary Cancer Prevention. McMaster University, Hamilton, Ontario, March 1999.

Farquhar, Andrew. "Exercising essentials." *Diabetes Dialogue*, Fall 1996; 43(3):6–8.

Ferraro, Cathleen. "New uses of chemicals linked to more illness." Scripps-McClatchy Western electronic news service, December 10, 1997.

"A Field Guide to Stress: A Conversation with Kenneth R. Pelletier, Ph.D." *Selfcare Archives*, December 15, 1997.

Fransen, Jenny and I. Jon Russell. *The Fibromyalgia Help Book*. St. Paul: Smith House Press, 1996.

Fredman, Catherine. "How to give a back rub." *Ladies Home Journal*, April 2000; 117(4):66.

Fugh-Berman, Adriane. *Alternative Medicine: What Works*. Tucson, AZ: Odonian Press, 1996.

"Get herbal relief." *Prevention*, July 1999; 51(7):128.

Getting to the Roots of a Vegetarian Diet. Baltimore: Vegetarian Resource Group, 1997.

Greenberg, Brigitte. "Stress hormone linked to high-fat snacking in women." The Associated Press Electronic news service, April 4, 1998.

Grout, Pam. "Tune out stress." *Ingram's*, April 1995; 21(4):78.

Gunawant, Deepika, and Gopi Warrier. *Ayurveda: The Ancient Indian Healing Tradition*. Shaftesbury, U.K.: Element, 1997.

Haas, Elson M. "Anti-stress nutritional program." HealthWorld Online. Retrieved from healthy.net, June 2000.

Hendler, Saul Sheldon. *The Doctors' Vitamin and Mineral Encyclopedia*. New York: Fireside Books, 1990.

Herring, Jeff. "Bring back passion to your everyday life." Knight Ridder/Tribune Electronic News Service, Feb 21, 2000 pK0535.

———. "Use these 10 tips to manage stress." Knight Ridder/Tribune Electronic News Service, Jan 31, 2000 pK0817.

———. "You can manage stress with HALTS." Knight-Ridder/Tribune Electronic News Service, May 22, 2000 pK1632.

Ho, Marian. "Learning your ABCs, part two." *Diabetes Dialogue*, Fall 1996; 43:3.

Hoffman, David L. "Herbal remedies and stress management." HealthWorld Online. Retrieved from healthy.net, June 2000.

———. "The nervous system and herbal remedies." HealthWorld Online. Retrieved from healthy.net, June 2000.

Hopson, Emma, and Judi Light Hopson. *Burnout to Balance: EMS Stress*. New York: Brady Books, 2000.

Hopson, Emma, Ted Hagen, and Judi Light Hopson. "Emotional support can help you cope with stress." Knight Ridder/Tribune Electronic News Service, August 30, 1999, pK7514.

"Hostility and heart risk." *Reuters Health Summary*, April 22, 1997.

"How forgiving helps you." *Redbook*, March 2000; 194(3):36.

"How to deal with stress." Retrieved from backrelief.com/stress.htm, February 12, 1999.

Hunt, Paula. "Touch up." *Vegetarian Times*, November 1999:96.

Iammetteo, Enzo. "The Alexander Technique: Improving the balance." *Performing Arts and Entertainment in Canada* Fall 1996; 30(3):37.

"Irritable bowel syndrome linked to emotional abuse." *Tufts University Health & Nutrition Letter*, April 2000; 18(2):3.

Jahnke, Roger. "Breathing practices." Healthy World Online. Retrieved from healthy.net, 2000.

———. *The Healer Within: The Four Essential Self-Care Methods for Creating Optimal Health*. New York: HarperCollins, 1997.

———. "Qigong." Healthy World Online. Retrieved from healthy.net, 2000.

———. "Self applied massage." Health World Online. Retrieved from healthy.net, 2000.

Joffe, Russell, and Anthony Levitt. *Conquering Depression*. Hamilton, Ontario: Empowering Press, 1998.

Johnson, Catherine. *When to Say Goodbye to Your Therapist*. New York: Simon and Schuster, 1988.

Johnson, Lois Joy. "You look divine: Stress management techniques." *Ladies Home Journal*, Jan 2000; 117(1):92.

Joplin, Janice. "The therapeutic benefits of expressive writing." *The Academy of Management Executive*, May 2000; 14(2):124.

Kaptchuk, Ted, and Michael Croucher. *The Healing Arts: A Journal Through the Faces of Medicine*. London: The British Broadcasting Corporation, 1986.

Kaslof, Leslie J. "Natural substances offer new hope for stress relief." HealthWorld Online. Retrieved from healthy.net, June 2000.

Keeping Women in Line [news segment]. Produced by *ABCNEWS 20/20*, originally aired July 21, 1995.

Keyishian, Amy. "Calming rituals for rotten days." *Cosmopolitan*, Feb 2000; 228(2):152.

"Kicking the habit: At last, a treatment that combats craving." *Scientific American*. Retrieved from sciam.com, January 2, 2000.

Kishi, Misa. *Impact of Pesticides on Health in Developing Countries: Research, Policy and Actions*. Paper presented at the World Conference on Breast Cancer, Kingston, Ontario, July13–17, 1997.

Kock, Henry. "Restoring natural vegetation as part of the farm." *Gardening without Chemicals '91*. Canadian Organic Growers Toronto Chapter, April 6, 1991.

Kotulak, Ronald. Researchers: Lack of sleep may cause aging, stress, flab. *Chicago Tribune*, April 5, 1998.

Kuczmarski, R.J., K.M. Flegal, S.M. Campbell, and C.L. Johnson. Increasing prevalence of overweight among U.S. adults: The National Health and Nutrition Examination surveys, 1960 to 1991. *Journal of the American Medical Association* 1994; 272:205–211.

Kushi, Mishio. *The Cancer Prevention Guide*. New York: St. Martin's Press, 1993.

Lad, Vasant. *Ayurveda: the Science of Self-Healing*. Santa Fe: Lotus Press, 1984.

Lark, Susan M. *Chronic Fatigue and Tiredness*. Los Altos, CA: Westchester Publishing Co., 1993.

Lemonick, Michael D. "Eat your heart out." *Time*, July 19, 1999.

Lippert Gray, Carol. *Get a Life.* Financial Executives Institute, 2000. Article A62599863.

Liu, Lynda. "A good cry." *Teen*, June 2000; 44(6):38.

Monhan Bartel, Margaret. "The woods in winter: Hiking as stress therapy." *Country Living*, Feb 1994; 17(2):65.

Mooy, Johanna M., Hendrik De Vries, Peter A. Grootenhuis, et al. "Major stressful life events in relation to prevalence of undetected type 2 diabetes." *Diabetes Care*, Feb 2000; 23(2):197.

Morrison, Judith H. *The Book of Ayurveda.* New York: Simon and Schuster, 1995.

Norment, Lynn. "Stress-busting secrets of superbusy people." *Ebony*, July 2000; 55(9):54.

Nyhout, Kristine. "Hands-on relief." *Chatelaine*, June 2000; 73(6):45.

Ontario Task Force on the Primary Prevention of Cancer. *Recommendations for the Primary Prevention of Cancer: Report of the Ontario Task Force on the Primary Prevention of Cancer.* Presented to the Ontario Ministry of Health, March 1995.

Canadian Diabetes Association. "Physical activity." *Equilibrium*, 1996; 1:22-23.

Pierpont, Margaret, and Diane Tegmeyer. *The Spa Life at Home.* Vancouver, B.C.: Whitecap Books, 1997.

Reing, Michael. "Stress and genital herpes recurrences in women." *Journal of the American Medical Association* 2000; 283(11):1394.

Rifkin, Jeremy. "Playing God with the genetic code." *Health Naturally* April/May 1995:40–44.

Roberts, Francine M. *The Therapy Sourcebook.* Chicago: NTC/Contemporary Publishing, 1998.

Rockett, Eva. "A passion for passion: How to live life at full throttle." *Canadian Living Health for Life*, Spring 2001.

Roizen, Michael F., and Elizabeth Anne Stephenson. *RealAge: Are You as Young as You Can Be?* New York: Cliff Street Books, 1999.

Rosen, Larry, and Michelle M. Weil. *Technostress: Coping With Technology@Work @Home @Play.* New York: John Wiley & Sons, 1997.

Rosenthal, M. Sara. *50 Ways to Manage Stress*. Chicago: McGraw-Hill, 2001.

———. *The Gastrointestinal Sourcebook*. Los Angeles: Lowell House, 1997.

———. *Managing Your Diabetes*. Toronto: Macmillan Canada, 1998.

———. *Women and Depression*. Chicago: NTC/Contemporary Publishing, 1999.

———. *Women and Passion*. Toronto: Prentice-Hall Canada, 2000.

———. *Women of the '60s Turning 50*. Toronto: Prentice-Hall Canada, 2000.

Rougher Arntz, Jane. "Under the gun? How you can cope with stress." *The Business Journal-Milwaukee* March 3, 2000; 17(23):18.

Seymour, Rhea. "Herpes alert." *Chatelaine*, Feb 2000; 73(2):46.

Shimer, Porter. *Keeping Fitness Simple: 500 Tips for Fitting Exercise into Your Life*. Pownal, VT: Storey Books, 1998.

Smereka, Corinne M. "Outwitting, controlling stress for a healthier lifestyle." *Healthcare Financial Management* March 1990; 44(3):70.

Smith, Sand. "Pulling your own strings: Three keys to personal power." *Office Solutions*, March 2000; 17(3):44.

Sobel, David. *Mental Medicine Update*, 1995, Vol IV, No. 3.

Spiker, Ted. "Choose to snooze." *Men's Health*, May 2000; 15(4):56.

"Stress affects your health more than you think." Posted to www.mediconsult.com, September 9, 1999.

"Stress may intensify cold symptoms." Posted to www.mediconsult.com, March 26, 1999.

"Stress-busters: What works." *Newsweek International*, June 28, 1999:52.

"Vacation of a lifetime." *Time*, March 20, 2000; 155(11):92.

Weed, Susun S. *Menopausal Years: The Wise Woman Way—Alternative Approaches for Women 30–90*. Woodstock, NY: Ash Tree Publishing, 1992.

———. *Wise Woman Ways: Menopausal Years*. Woodstock, NY: Ash Tree Publishing, 1992.

Weintraub, Amy. "The natural Prozac." Health World Online.
    Retrieved from healthy.net, 2000.

"Writing about stress improves your health." *Research Digest.*
    Retrieved from mediconsult.com, June 16, 1999.

Zand, Janet. "Herbal programs for stress." HealthWorld Online.
    Retrieved from healthy.net, June 2000.

Zellerbach, Merla. *The Allergy Sourcebook*. Los Angeles: Lowell House,
    1995.

Index